CHRONIC

CHRONIC

CHRISTINE M. RICH

NEW DEGREE PRESS

CHRONIC

ISBN   978-1-63676-482-5   *Paperback*

            978-1-63730-387-0   *Kindle Ebook*

            978-1-63730-388-7   *Ebook*

For my best friend and greatest teacher, Joe. Twenty years later you still make me swoon.

For my sweet little fairies, Stella and Roma. I am in awe of you both every single day.

And for the 80 percent ... you will never be invisible to me.

CONTENTS

————

"*And I said to my body softly, 'I want to be your friend.' It took a long breath and replied, 'I have been waiting my whole life for this.'*"

-NAYYIRAH WAHEED

NOTE FROM THE AUTHOR

———

As a child, I always loved reading and knew one day I wanted to write a book. Initially, I thought I should write about women in leadership—a project I hoped would inspire other women and look impressive on my resume.

This is not that book—because a different story kept calling to me, try as I might to ignore it.

My own.

This is the book I needed to write, even though I felt terrified to share such personal details in print—that people might *actually* read. For years I carried a secret. Despite how confident and together I looked on the outside, on the inside, I often felt afraid and angry as I struggled to accept what it meant to live with an invisible disease. One that no amount of perceived "togetherness" would cure.

The word "chronic" is often associated with long-term, negative things like illness and pain. (Although, I've often wondered why we don't use the term to describe positive things like love and wellness.) Autoimmune diseases typically fall into the negative-chronic category.

According to the National Institutes of Health, *autoimmune disease* is a condition in which the immune system mistakenly attacks the body, creating inflammation and disease. There are an estimated one hundred different types, and roughly 80 percent of people with an autoimmune disease in the US are women. I am one of those women with one of those autoimmune diseases called Crohn's—and this is my story.

Chronic is the book I wish would have existed when I was a teenager, struggling to process and accept my diagnosis, and later as a young wife, mother, and professional with a chronic illness. For years, I did not understand the emotional impact the term "chronic" had on me; and I carried so much guilt for feeling anything other than grateful. I thought my disease was something I could simply run away from, sweep under the rug, fight against, or achieve my way out of.

Spoiler alert: none of those things worked. By pushing against my body and all of the emotional and mental struggles that accompany living with Crohn's disease, I was denying and fighting against myself and, most importantly, my spirit. Which was no way to live the wholehearted life I wanted.

Crohn's disease can be a tough one, especially for women living in a society that expects them to be pretty, neat, and appeasing at all times. "Ladylike" is a term I heard a lot growing up. Guess what is not particularly ladylike? Pretty much all the main symptoms of Crohn's disease! After all, women aren't supposed to be gassy, have diarrhea, or shit themselves in the middle of the workday. And heaven forbid we actually talk about such things out loud! We're also not supposed to be too emotional (especially not angry) or too demanding about what we need.

Many of us were taught to smile, be grateful, and make everyone else feel all comfy cozy at the expense of our own comfort and well-being. The problem with these types of expectations is that they are lies that create shame, loneliness, and rage that eventually turn women against themselves and their potential. In my experience, these lies lead to one of two places: an eventual brick wall we run straight into, going one hundred miles per hour, or worse, a nagging feeling we are meant for more but are too afraid to show up for fear of being truly seen.

Like anyone else, I made mistakes and decisions of which I'm not proud. I made an enemy of my body and took it for granted for years. I refused to listen to or trust myself, even when a small voice inside was begging me to. And I lived in a perpetual state of fight-or-flight until I learned another way.

It wasn't until my body waved the white flag and started shutting down that I realized I had to make a decision: I could continue on the path of denial and destruction, or I could learn to accept, love, and listen to my body in order to become the woman I was meant to be. The good news is, as Glinda said in *The Wizard of Oz*, I had the power all along. And so do you.

My hope for this book is to help other women who are living with any kind of chronic condition feel less alone and more validated. I want to create a space for you, the reader, to reflect on everything you've been through. The good, the bad, the embarrassing, whatever. That's why I've included journal prompts at the end of each section in this book. I hope you will take the time to write and reflect as you discover new things about yourself and your experiences.

I also hope that this book serves as a tool to help all women feel empowered to grieve, feel, ask for help, tell the truth, and advocate for and take care of their bodies and spirits. This is not a story about overcoming a monster or slaying a dragon because that would only result in fighting against ourselves. (And something tells me if you're reading this book and have a chronic issue, you've done enough of that already.) This is a story about befriending ourselves—especially the parts that scare us or are what others might consider broken or different.

As it turns out, I not only needed to write this book for myself, but also for other women who might be struggling. There is power in sharing our stories, however messy, raw, and "un-resume-worthy" they might be. Ultimately, this is a book for anyone who has ever struggled with self-acceptance in whatever form that may take. For me, it is Crohn's disease—for you, it might be a different autoimmune disease, addiction, or a physical disability. Here's what I know for sure—we all carry *something*, and my hope is this book will help lighten your load just a little.

Chronically yours,
Christine

PART 1

FREEZING

CHAPTER 1

DRESSES

Ever since I was a little girl, I have always loved dresses. They're quick and easy, and I always feel pulled together and— let's face it—*noticed* in a dress.

My penchant for dress-wearing started young. There was the empire-waist Cabbage Patch number I wore to my fifth birthday party. The red fit-and-flare dress my aunt bought me when I was nine that floated around me when I spun, just like Penny in *Dirty Dancing*. There were the obvious ones like the head-to-toe teal sequins gown I wore to prom my junior year (with dyed matching shoes, thank you very much!) and, of course, my wedding dress.

What I realized from a relatively young age is that a dress can be a pretty slick veneer—a costume, a way to present oneself to the world as the kind of girl who is sweet and cute or the kind of woman who is confident and put together.

Just like those women who look like they just stepped out of *InStyle* magazine on early-morning flights. *Who are these fancy airport women?* How did they manage to pull off hair, makeup, and all that chicness for a 6 a.m. flight? As a kid, I would secretly admire these types of women and dreamed of the day when I too could be a fancy airport woman. And then I became one and realized it wasn't all that fancy. After all, there's nothing fancy about living in a constant state of fear, anger, and denial. And dress or no dress, there is certainly nothing fancy about losing control of one's bodily functions in the middle of a workday. Or maybe there is—if such moments serve as wake-up calls.

One such moment involved a little black dress (LBD) with just the right amount of stretch and perfectly placed pockets. An LBD with stretch *and* pockets is like the holy grail of dresses. And this one was comfortable, classic, could be crumpled up in a ball and still be ready to wear within a moment's notice. I loved and wore the hell out of that dress for years.

It also happened to be the dress I was wearing when I shit myself—a very common, not often discussed reality of living with Crohn's disease.

In the middle of a workday.

In a fairly crowded Hilton parking lot. (Mortifying!)

On a hot summer day wearing open-toed heels. (You do the math.)

Fancy dress and all.

The desecration of my favorite LBD happened the day before I was admitted to the hospital, where I would spend a week finally coming to terms with a diagnosis I had been running away from for years. I was twenty-nine years old and never learned how to properly care for my Crohn's-ravaged body and, perhaps more importantly, my broken spirit. (More on this humiliating, life-changing experience later.)

The second life-changing-dress-moment happened years later, while I was wearing a red Calvin Klein shift that fit like a glove. (Those fancy airport women would have approved!) It was the day of a big work presentation; I wore red because it was the color of our company logo, and I wanted to be "on brand" when I made my big pitch. I was prepared and ready to present with the ease of a strong, confident, professional woman.

For some reason, I also thought it was a brilliant idea to cram in a quick therapy sesh ... three hours before my presentation.

Did I mention my therapist specializes in *trauma healing*?

The week prior, I sat across from my therapist, Koren, and confessed I felt like my insides didn't match my outsides. I was simultaneously jittery and exhausted the majority of the time. There was unsettled energy coursing through my veins, living just beneath the surface. She suggested I had some pent-up anger, handed me a piece of rubber hose, and invited me to hit the small punching bag she kept in her office.

Um ... you want me to do what? No fucking way am I hitting that bag. How ridiculous! I'm not angry. I'm just a workaholic.

"No thank you," I smiled and politely declined.

I was thinking about that interaction on the drive to that afternoon's therapy appointment when I called my husband, Joe. "I know she's going to try to get me to hit that stupid bag."

"So hit the bag, Chris." He made it sound so easy.

"I mean, I want to ... I really do. I just don't think I'm physically able to. It's like I can't let go or something." I fidgeted with the radio while cradling the phone between my ear and shoulder.

He suggested that maybe what I needed most was someone to witness my pain. To sit with me while I processed and let it out. Joe always seemed to know what I needed before I did.

And maybe he was right. Maybe I was in pain and needed someone to witness all of my ugly, hot, "unladylike" rage. Maybe I needed to see it too.

Then I showed up to my appointment all prim and proper and instantly started talking myself out of this whole business of "needing a witness." I mean, what would it solve anyway? It's not like I was going to tap some lame punching bag and all of a sudden feel better.

I sat down on the couch across from my therapist and secretly hoped she wouldn't bring it up. Maybe she forgot about my anger and anxiety, and we could have a nice, civilized chat for the next fifty minutes.

No such luck.

Within the first five minutes, she pulled out the punching bag. "Do you want to try releasing some of that emotion?" She handed me the hose and nodded toward the bag. Resistance started burning in my chest.

Then I heard Joe's words ringing in my mind:

A witness. I need a witness. Let her be that witness.

"Sure, okay." I took a breath and grabbed the hose. I stood up, smoothed out my red Calvin Klein dress, and gently tapped the bag, feeling self-conscious.

"Okay good. Now hit it harder and let out a deep breath. You don't need to hold back in here." Koren watched me with her hands folded in her lap as if a grown woman hitting a punching bag was the most normal thing in the world to observe.

No need to hold back. What an unusual concept. I trained myself to hold back all of my big, uncomfortable feelings for so long. It was time to let go. It was clear these feelings

weren't serving me, and they sure as hell weren't going anywhere anytime soon. *A witness. Let her witness you ... even
if it's raw and messy.*

After a few whacks, I actually started to get into it and
allowed myself to let go. Red dress and all. I felt uncomfortable and ridiculous at first, but then something started to
happen—I started to *feel*.

I hit the bag harder and harder as I began to access feelings that were buried inside me for years.

Whack!

"Good, now hit it again and tell me what you're feeling."

"I'm ... I'm mad? I think ..." *Whack!*

"No ... I'm actually *more* than mad." *Whack!* I began to
feel the self-consciousness leave my body.

"I'm PISSED!" *Whack!*

"Good! Yes! You have every right to be." Her voice
remained calm and soothing.

Whack! Whack! Whack!

"Now breathe. Really let it out every time you hit the bag."
She suggested I try yelling out loud each time I hit the bag.

I stopped momentarily and looked at her like she was
insane.

Koren leaned in as if to tell me a secret, "No one's in the
office but you and me." She could sense my self-consciousness returning and wanted to reassure me I was safe—a feeling I'd been chasing for decades.

So, I closed my eyes, took a breath, and finally let go.

I beat the living hell out of that punching bag for the next
two minutes, making loud grunting noises with each hit. The
harder I hit, the louder the grunts. The louder the grunts,
the harder I hit. I started sweating and could feel what was
bubbling beneath the surface starting to break up.

Whack! Whack! Whack!

I lost control in the best way possible and eventually broke down sobbing. Tears, snot, and sweat covered my dress—and I never felt more free or beautiful in my entire life.

I've heard therapists say that anger is a secondary emotion: the "bodyguard of sadness." In that moment, I finally understood firsthand the truth in that statement. Because behind the fancy-airport-woman façade, behind the smiles and each carefully selected dress, was a sad and grieving girl in need of love and care.

Both "dress scenarios" were major a-ha moments in my life. You see, I used to be pretty stubborn and preferred to keep busy in order to avoid all the things I didn't want to feel. Classic stress response cycle ... good old flight, fight, or freeze—not a great strategy, and one I desperately needed to unlearn. It wasn't until I ran into a few brick walls that I was finally able to see what a mess of things I had made.

I used to be a major "brick wall" kinda gal. Brick walls taught me a lot about loving myself enough to slow down and treat my body like a friend instead of an enemy just because it happens to be different. But a woman can only run into so many brick walls before they crush her. The trick is not to let them form in the first place, which is a hell of a lot easier said than done.

It helps to remember who we were and what we wanted before we felt the need to hide behind fancy dresses, facades, and brick walls.

"Tears, snot, and sweat covered my dress—and I never felt more free or beautiful in my entire life."

CHAPTER 2

NERVOUS NELLY

———

I was recently interviewed on my friend Shannon's podcast *Rule Breaker by Rebelle*. The first question she asked me was what I wanted to become when I was a little girl. I smiled, thinking back to my childhood bedroom where I would play house. But not my house, Angela Bower's house.

You remember Angela Bower ... from the 1980s sitcom *Who's the Boss*. If you're too young to know about *Who's the Boss* or have simply forgotten about one of the greatest female characters of all time, allow me to refresh your memory.

Angela Bower was an advertising executive, single mom, and eventual business owner (she started her own agency after being fired for losing a client for essentially taking a vacation!). She had phenomenally frosted hair and wore the most incredible suits and colorful dresses with shoulder pads the size of Big Macs. Angela was my idol because she was the first woman I ever saw who was:

    a) A total boss babe

    b) A mom

c) Confidently rocked both roles with a little help from her hottie-with-a-body housekeeper, Tony Micelli. (I have always loved an Italian man who can cook and clean!)

My version of "house" always starred me as a working mom with an adorable baby I lovingly carried on my hip throughout the workday. Sometimes I was an ad executive like Angela. Other times I was a writer like my favorite author Judy Blume. Once, I was even a backup dancer for this new artist named Mariah Carey.

I thought if Angela Bower could do both, why couldn't I? I also spent time in my bedroom playing dress-up, writing poems, organizing my caboodle filled with teal-and-pink Wet n Wild eyeshadow, and daydreaming about the big, beautiful life I would have for myself someday.

As bold and brave as I felt inside my bedroom, the world outside of it often felt like a big, scary place. Although I learned to hide my fears and anxieties behind a big smile and energetic personality, I lived with an extensive list of highly unlikely fears and phobias.

Let's see, there was the summer I was terrified of getting Lyme disease and refused to play in any grass taller than my ankle for fear of killer ticks. (Keep in mind, I had no idea what Lyme disease actually was. I just knew it was something to fear.)

In fifth grade, I was afraid of getting possessed by the devil after watching a 20/20 episode where Barbara Walters interviewed a girl who experienced a real-life possession. I'm not sure if this was a Catholic thing or just a generalized anxiety thing, but nonetheless, I was terrified and certain it would happen to me.

I was also afraid of tornados, lead poisoning, raw oysters ... pretty much anything that could result in an untimely death.

1987

My nervousness started in first grade with an irrational fear of the woods near my elementary school. One evening, during dinner, my dad mentioned something about people illegally hunting in the woods behind my school. The only thing my tender little seven-year-old brain heard was "men with guns," and I instantly felt afraid and unsafe—so much so that I found every excuse not to go outside for recess, for fear of being picked off by one of the raging lunatic snipers hiding out in the woods. My stomach hurt the moment I thought of those woods.

I also found it really odd that no one else shared my concern.

My teacher, clearly oblivious to the looming danger, would enthusiastically announce it was time to get ready for recess.

Nice try, lady. There is no way I'm going within striking distance of those woods. I don't care how freshly painted the hopscotch board is ... not a chance in hell.

This went on for about a week. Until one day, my mother quietly snuck into my classroom, whispered something to my teacher, and then knelt beside my desk. "Come on Chris, grab your coat. We're going on a little field trip."

A field trip? In the middle of a school day! I was beyond excited.

On our way out of the classroom, I imagined where she was taking me. I envisioned a trip to Hills to buy a cherry slush and a sleeve of salty popcorn. Maybe if I was lucky, I would even score the new Peaches n' Cream Barbie I'd been eyeing for weeks.

Instead of walking to the car, she veered toward the woods outside my classroom. "Mom, where are we going?" I started to panic because I already knew the answer.

"Into the woods." Her tone was calm and matter-of-fact.

"What? No! There are bad guys with guns! No mommy, please! We can't! It's not safe!"

"Chris, do you think I would ever put you in harm's way? We are going into these woods together and I will show you there is nothing to be scared of." She grabbed my hand and led the way.

Fear washed over me. I held on to my mother for dear life and squeezed my eyes shut.

"Open your eyes. You'll see, there's nothing to be afraid of." She spoke softly but confidently. I slowly opened my eyes, terrified of what I would see.

"Look around, Chris. There's nothing here that will hurt you."

I vigilantly scanned my surroundings, waiting for a pack of gun-crazed men to attack. As my eyes adjusted and we kept going deeper into the woods, I realized it was actually quite beautiful and felt my body begin to relax.

Along the way, we talked and picked up litter: an old Mountain Dew can, some crumpled paper, and fast-food bags. At that moment, my mom became my hero.

When we finally returned to the classroom, everyone was getting their coats on for recess and gathered around me excitedly. "Where did you go?"

My mom hugged me and gave me a little wink on her way out.

"I went into the woods." I smiled shyly. My classmates looked at me, slightly disappointed—but I was not.

Facing my fears by walking into the woods was a great lesson. The longer I avoided going out to recess, the stronger my fear grew. That day I learned it was possible to be afraid and brave at the same time and to see the beauty and truth that fear often masks.

But let's be clear: my anxiety was not magically cured with one walk in the woods. It ebbed and flowed throughout my childhood and became the perfect alibi for my ongoing digestive issues.

* * *

From a young age, I used to get really bad stomachaches. I'd be outside playing with friends one minute, and before I could even lay claim to my make-believe boyfriend, Mike Seaver (you know, ... the dreamy big brother from *Growing Pains*), my body would break out in chills, and I'd be doubled over in pain.

Eventually, I'd have to hop on my pink-and-purple Huffy bike, pedal home as fast as I could, and run straight to the bathroom. By the time I returned to my friends, everyone had moved on to a new game. That's just the way it was for me and my stomach. My family expected that wherever we went, eventually, I'd have to use the bathroom. This phenomenon carried into my teenage years and progressively got worse.

1996–1997

The summer before my junior year of high school, I went on vacation with my two best friends, and we'd laugh about how neither one of them had ever known anyone who pooped as much as I did. "Every time you eat anything you have to run immediately to the bathroom," they laughed.

"I know, it's kind of amazing," I'd say, trying to downplay. "I mean, I can eat whatever I want and not gain a pound!"

But secretly, I was starting to get worried. It didn't seem right to have to use the bathroom so often. I even started to notice a little bit of blood every now and then. I dismissed it as a "nervous stomach" and didn't say much to my parents because I figured it would just resolve itself and go away on its own. Not a great strategy.

By the following year, things started to change. My stomach hurt all the time, and I pretty much couldn't eat anything without immediately getting sick. As a sixteen-year-old girl, it was mortifying to have to go to the bathroom all the time. It was around this time that I also started noticing whole, undigested food in the toilet—along with a lot more blood. Which was startling and scary, to say the least.

I also started losing weight but receiving a lot of praise for it. As a young girl who grew up during the '90s supermodel era, in my mind, this was awesome. The skinnier I got, the more attention I got. Even more than when I would wear a dress. And as sad as it sounds, I secretly loved it.

At the time, I was convinced that—unlike my friends, who had all sorts of talents and abilities—the only thing it felt like I ever got attention for was how I looked. And everyone was telling me how great I looked, so I figured it wasn't all that bad. I continued to keep quiet about how I was feeling and what was really going on. Looking back, this was the beginning of my lifelong battle with body dysmorphia. I could either feel sick and be rail-thin or feel healthy and be a normal size. Sadly, in those days and many years after, I prioritized being sick and thin.

Then crippling fatigue started to kick in. Not the average teenage tiredness, but an all-consuming exhaustion that made me feel like I never slept the night before. The kind of fatigue that is physically painful and impossible to deny. I would fall asleep in class, nap when I got home from school—for hours on end—and was always the first to fall asleep at sleepovers, resulting in many frozen bras (the classic teenage-girl consequence for falling asleep first).

Fatigue. How does one accurately explain the difference between being tired versus being *autoimmune disease tired*? Natalie Hayden—fellow Crohn's warrior and friend—wrote a piece on her blog *Lights, Camera, Crohn's* in October 2020, asking her readers to help describe what this type of fatigue feels like. Here are a few of my favorite responses:

"Knowing I need to walk 100 feet to get to my work building and having to give myself a pep talk to do it because I'm not sure I'll make it without having to sit down." *Ah, yes.*

"Like you're walking with ankle and wrist weights on 24/7." *And a weighted vest.*

"When I think of chronic fatigue for me it means faking being well. No matter how much sleep you get, you still wake up tired. Chronic illness fatigue is physical, mental, and emotional exhaustion." *Check! Check! And check!*

"Down to the bone, exhaustion in my core, something that is impossible to push through." *But we do anyway.*

"Heaviness in my body. Just surviving, not thriving. Frustrating, because I want to do more things but can't." *So much frustration.*

For me, the fatigue felt like walking uphill … in mud … carrying two soaking-wet weighted blankets on my back … in the rain. Walking down the halls of my school felt like climbing Mount Everest, but I did it every day and with a smile on my face. Despite how badly I felt, I continued to go out with my friends and work at my part-time job. I was involved in activities, got good grades, went to basketball games, and had sleepovers.

Not putting two and two together, I figured I was out of shape and decided it was time to start working out on top of everything else. I pushed my body when what it needed most was rest—a habit I would need to unlearn as I got older. My mom noticed things getting worse and started hounding me to go to the doctor. I didn't want to hear it. Looking back, this was when I started hiding. I told her it was "no big deal," but inside, I knew better—and I was terrified.

Eventually, my mom took me to our family doctor. To say I wasn't happy about it is an understatement. I didn't want to go or talk about what was happening. I just wanted to close my eyes, plug my ears like a petulant child, and wait for everything to go away on its own.

The moment the doctor came into the room, my mom started rattling off a list of all my symptoms. The frequent trips to the bathroom, the blood, the pain and exhaustion, the weight loss. Sitting on the exam table, I felt mortified when I was asked to explain, in painstaking detail, the exact consistency of my bowel movements. I was so mad at my mom for putting me through this humiliation. I could feel my face turning red and wanted to crawl under a rock.

"Oh, …" my mom chimed in, "… and it smells like toxic waste." I thought I might actually die right then and there.

The doctor looked me over, listened to my heart, and pressed on my stomach once. She didn't seem remotely fazed or concerned when she told my mom I was probably just a nervous kid with a nervous stomach. "From what I recall, she's always been a bit of a perfectionist."

I was confused. Was that supposed to be a formal diagnosis? The last time I checked, perfectionism didn't make people shit blood, double over with pain, and cause extreme exhaustion. As much as I didn't want to be there, I felt confused by my doctor's assessment. But what did I know? I was just a sixteen-year-old girl who was taught to respect and not question authority figures. So that's exactly what I did. I figured a doctor who saw me once a year knew better than I did about what I was experiencing.

Try as I might to hide my symptoms from my parents, my mama wasn't having it. We went back to the same doctor a month later because things were getting worse, and I'd lost even more weight. Truth be told, I was starting to get a little worried.

This time around, my doctor seemed genuinely annoyed to see us again, and conceded to giving me a rectal exam (WITH MY MOTHER IN THE ROOM!). They then suggested I likely had a case of perfectionism *and* hemorrhoids. I wanted to die right then and there. What teenage girl has hemorrhoids?

My mom refused to be blown off a second time and insisted there must be some kind of test to be sure it wasn't something more serious. Eventually, the doctor reluctantly ordered a diagnostic procedure called a barium enema.

"I highly doubt anything will come back wrong, but we can do this test if it makes you feel better," the doctor hissed, without so much as a glance in my direction.

We thanked her—for what, I'm not sure. I got dressed and felt worse than when I arrived. I felt like I had offended my doctor and started second-guessing myself. Maybe it wasn't all that bad. Maybe I was making a mountain out of a bloody molehill. Maybe I was crazy?

All I wanted to do was go home, crawl in bed, put the whole "finger-up-my-butt-thing" behind me, and get ready for my test. Whatever a *barium enema* was, it didn't sound so bad, and I just wanted some answers.

I should probably note here that no one explained to me or my mother what happened during the barium enema prep or procedure. Nor did anyone warn me that the doctor who performed the procedure would end up looking like George *Fricking* Clooney from his days as Dr. Doug Ross on *ER*. It felt like there was no end to the level of embarrassment I was being subjected to.

Long story short, the test came back as inconclusive. We were back to square one. Was the pain, diarrhea, blood, mucous, and exhaustion really just all in my head? Maybe this was just the way my body was going to be from now on. After all, I had some good days every now and then. There wasn't *always* blood when I went to the bathroom. Sometimes I was able to eat and not sprint to the nearest bathroom. Maybe I just needed to toughen up and learn to live with the pain.

Here's the thing I didn't know then or even a decade after my diagnosis: the body doesn't lie. It speaks to us. It tells us what it needs and sends us signals when something is off. But it requires trusting ourselves enough to listen, advocate, and insist we keep working to find an answer—even if a doctor gets annoyed.

Especially if a doctor gets annoyed.

And in case you're a recovering people pleaser like I was for years, allow me to share some advice. You have the right to know exactly what is going to happen to your body. You have every right to clear explanations and clarifications without feeling like you're *bothering* your doctor. You have every right to say, "I don't understand. Can you please explain this to me another way?" or "I'm not comfortable with that plan ... what else you got?"

What I really needed to do was channel my inner Angela Bower, but I didn't exactly know how ... yet.

*"I learned to hide
my fears and
anxieties behind
a big smile and
energetic personality."*

CHAPTER 3

CUJO

During my sophomore year in high school, there was a girl, a grade behind me, who died of stomach cancer. She deteriorated so quickly, and it was a shock to everyone. I couldn't stop thinking about her and wondered if the same thing would happen to me. Was my doctor overlooking something? How could the barium enema come back inconclusive if I still felt sick and was clearly getting worse? I tried to push those thoughts out of my mind, but try as I might, there was no running away from the symptoms.

I was afraid to know what was really going on and even more terrified of never finding out. By the time school started in the fall of my senior year, things had gotten much worse. My exhaustion intensified, the constant and sudden urge to use the bathroom intensified, the blood and pain intensified. I tried so hard to ignore or downplay my symptoms in the hopes they would magically disappear. I simply did not want to deal with any of it.

In order to manage day-to-day, I had to disconnect from my body just to function. Looking back, I can see this was my first lesson in abandoning my body to avoid pain and fear. But in all fairness, it felt like my body was abandoning me.

Every time I ate, I would get waves of nausea and sharp pains in my stomach that would make me double over in pain and break out in goosebumps all over my body. I didn't want to let on to anyone just how bad it was, so I learned to breathe through the pain and either stay really still until it passed, or I could rush to the nearest bathroom and get sick. Every day felt like a battle I was slowly losing.

After every episode—which went from being a few-times-a-week situation to an all-day, everyday nightmare—I would feel completely emptied and hollowed out. Like every last bit of joy, energy, and life was being violently sucked out of my body and flushed down the toilet. I would come out of the bathroom feeling dizzy, weak, and defeated. At that time, I made all sorts of deals with God.

Please just let me get better, and I swear I will be a good person. I'm so sorry for all of my sins.

Please take this from me because I can't do this much longer. I'm so sorry for whatever I did to cause this.

I swear I'll change ... please heal me. I don't want to die.

In the end, no amount of prayers, naps, or special diets helped. I was simply not getting better and couldn't quite shake the feeling of being punished for something.

I would wake up after sleeping for twelve hours and feel like I never slept. I was freezing all the time. My periods became extremely irregular. My eyes were sunken, and every day I piled on blush just to give my skin some sort of color other than gray.

The strange part was, even though I felt like holy hell, people would often tell me—no, *praise* me—over and over for how skinny I looked. How *lucky* I was to be so skinny. How they *wished* they were as small as me. The sicker I became, the thinner I became, and the thinner I became, the more compliments and praise I received, which did a real number on my body image. I felt like I was expected to stay a size two for all eternity because that was the size people seemed to love me most at.

After a while, I figured out how easy and superficial it was to hide just how bad I felt. Here's the drill: Put on a casual dress but don't show too much skin ... they'll see just how skinny you've become. No matter how tired you are, do your hair and makeup. A little mascara, concealer, blush, and lipstick and one can pass for a perfectly healthy, together human being.

In our warped society, the standard of beauty is the thinner, the better; and as long as you're wearing lipstick, you must be A-OK. In 2017, Pew Research conducted a study on gender differences. The study asked 4,573 adults what they thought society valued in each gender. For men, the number-one valued characteristic was honesty & morality. Can you guess what the number-one characteristic was for women? Physical attractiveness.

This is why so many autoimmune diseases and chronic illnesses are referred to as "invisible." No one could tell I was sick just by looking at me—especially when I hid behind perceived "physical attractiveness." And just like I hid my anxiety as a kid, I hid my failing health as long as I could. But my mom knew better and refused to let up until we had an answer. No amount of make-up was fooling her.

Eventually, in November, I was referred to a gastroenterologist: a handsome man in his early fifties who had pretty blue eyes and looked like the baseball player Cal Ripken, Jr. He performed a colonoscopy, which is a procedure where a long, flexible tube is inserted into the rectum with a tiny video camera at the tip. It's like a GoPro for your poop shoot.

The rectal GoPro gets snaked through the entire colon, looking for abnormalities like inflammation, polyps, and cancer. Sedation, or "twilight," as it's sometimes referred to, is typically required because it's not the most comfortable procedure in the world.

After the colonoscopy, my father carried my frail, sedated body from the car into the house like a small child. I slept for the rest of the afternoon until I woke up groggy and starving from not eating in nearly forty-eight hours due to the prep required. The "prep" involves no solid foods for twenty-four hours prior to the procedure, alongside a nasty drink that tastes like death and makes you shit water until your colon is squeaky-clean and ready for primetime. I was just shy of eighteen years old, and in the course of a few months, I'd had more strangers stick more objects up my butt than I ever imagined was possible.

A few days later, we were called back to my new doctor's office.

What I didn't realize then, that I fully realize now, is that when you get any kind of medical test, if nothing is wrong, they don't bring you into the office to tell you your results. They tell you right away on the phone. BAM! You're fine. Or the old adage "no news is good news." Clearly, there was news to share.

The morning of my follow-up appointment, my parents and I were ushered into an examination room by a nurse and eagerly awaited the doctor. The nurse handed something to my parents before she left the room. By that point, I was so worn out and tired I just wanted answers. Anyone who has a chronic illness knows the saying all too well—I was so sick and tired of being so sick and tired.

I could tell my parents were anxious. My mother was obsessively clearing her throat and nostrils (a sound that, to this day, makes me cringe). Meanwhile, my father was bouncing his knee, chewing his fingernails, and nervously smiling at me—then looking away.

I was staring straight ahead at a print hanging on the wall across from the examination table. It was one of those cheesy motivational posters that were really big in the '90s. There were all sorts of them.

SUCCESS.

"Some people dream of success ... while others wake up and work hard at it."

ASPIRE.

"You will become as small as your controlling desire; as great as your dominant aspiration."

PERSPECTIVE.

"If you change the way you view the path, the path itself will change."

While I can't remember the theme of the poster that was hanging in the examination room, I do remember the image: a man on top of a cold, snowy mountain—all alone. He looked so small with the mountain beneath him and the crystal blue sky all around him. He had done it. He conquered the insurmountable mountain. He made it and was taking in all the beauty and majesty that surrounded him.

The word was probably something like JOURNEY or PERSEVERANCE. I smiled to myself, temporarily forgot where I was, and imagined all the mountains I would conquer when I went to college next year.

I glanced over at my parents, and my smile quickly faded as I saw their faces. "What's wrong?"

They looked at each other with wide eyes and then down at a videotape the nurse had handed my mom.

"What? What is it?" I could feel the energy in the room shift, and it annoyed me.

My mom smiled awkwardly and, with tears in her eyes, flashed me the cover of the videotape: "Living with Crohn's."

Crohn's. Crohn's? What is that? I've heard of it before. But where?

"Why would the nurse give you that before we saw the doctor? Wait, what is Crohn's? Don't we know someone who has it?" I could hear my heart beating in my ears.

My dad shook his head but kept his eyes locked on the floor. "Ya, we do. My old boss's daughter. She has Crohn's. Remember? You used to play with her when you were little." I could hear his voice starting to shake ever so slightly. It made me uncomfortable because the only time I ever saw my dad get emotional was at his father's funeral.

"Wait—that's what she had? Wasn't she always really sick? Didn't she have to have, like, multiple surgeries? Aren't there a lot of complications with it?" I started flashing back to a beautiful but fragile little girl with strawberry blonde hair who I was told might not live as long as other people. My throat started tightening.

Before my dad had a chance to answer me, the doctor came into the room.

I instantly felt hot, and my stomach started hurting in a way that was so much worse than it typically did. This was a different kind of pain; it stretched from my gut all the way up to my chest and throat. My breath became shallow, and my skin felt tingly all over.

The doctor confirmed what the tape said: I was, in fact, living with Crohn's. He explained that Crohn's is an inflammatory bowel disease (IBD) that causes inflammation along the digestive tract. "Anywhere from the mouth to the anus." He likened it to having strep throat in my colon (how's that for a visual?)

He said words like fistula, bowel obstruction, colon cancer, and anal fissures. He spoke of additional tests, more bloodwork, and stool samples. Nothing he said made any sense, and it felt like someone was slowly dimming a light inside me.

My mom instantly started crying. My dad bounced his knee even harder. Everyone was watching me, and I felt both stunned and guilty for causing them so much pain. My guilt quickly turned to irritation at my mom for openly sobbing after the doctor confirmed that there was, in fact, "no cure."

My parents had their go-to reactions in times of high stress. Typically, my mom would go into emotional overload and worst-case scenario mode, which made my dad—who grew up in the Archie Bunker generation of "men don't cry"— super uncomfortable and mad. Which, in turn, made my mom more emotional. Which, in turn, made my dad angrier.

Which, in turn, made me shut down and retreat inward to avoid all of it.

"Chrissy ... do you understand what I'm saying to you? Do you understand what this means?" The doctor's voice was gentle and kind. I looked over at the poster of the man alone on the mountain, refusing to make eye contact with him. "Chris?"

My eyes shifted away from the poster to the three adults in the room. I felt anger course through my veins. I wanted to rip that goddamn picture off the wall and smash it over my doctor's head. I wanted to scream at my mother to stop crying like a fucking baby, and I wanted to punch my dad in the leg to make him stop shaking it. I felt them all staring at me, pitying me, waiting for me to say something or react. But I didn't dare make a move.

Instead, I did the only thing I could think of, which was to make everyone else feel comfortable—my go-to reaction in times of high stress. It was the role I was used to playing, and I was really good at it. So, I took a deep breath, swallowed every single negative emotion I was feeling, and smiled.

"Yes, I understand. It's fine. I'm fine." And with that lie, a small lump formed in my throat. "Is there anything else or can we go?"

* * *

When I was little, the first scary movie my parents let me watch was Stephen King's *Cujo*, about a rabid dog hell-bent on killing a mother and her son stuck in a broken-down car. Throughout the movie, they tried desperately to get to the house for safety—but Cujo blocked their path and wouldn't let them through.

That's what fear felt like to me at that moment: like a big, scary, rabid dog growling and showing his teeth about to devour me whole. I thought, if I don't make any sudden moves, don't make direct eye contact, just smile and slowly back away, everything will be fine.

That feeling … that fear of being attacked and torn to shreds … stayed with me for years. In the beginning, I froze, never really taking a full inhale or exhale for fear of disturbing the beast. Then I tried running, but that damn dog would chase after me. He was always hot on my trail, watching me, ready to launch into an attack at any moment. Eventually, I tried fighting, but that didn't work either.

It would take me years and several failed attempts at freezing, flying, and fighting in order to realize what I really needed was to stop turning my disease—and ultimately myself—into a monster. There was a fourth "F" I needed to learn:

Friendship.

But I was nowhere near ready to make friends with my chronic illness because you can't befriend something you're afraid of and unwilling to accept. I needed to go into the woods like I did when I was a scared first grader but wasn't even sure how to get there. So, I avoided that terrifying place at all costs.

"Nothing he said made any sense, and it felt like someone was slowly dimming a light inside me."

CHAPTER 4

JAGGED LITTLE PILLS

———

Walking into my doctor's office the morning of my diagnosis, I naively thought I was prepared for whatever I was about to learn. Walking out a mere hour later with my parents, I felt numb as I carried a folder full of pamphlets and a handful of prescriptions with me to the car.

As for the "Living with Crohn's" videotape, my mom snagged it on our way out because I refused to acknowledge its existence. And there wasn't a snowball's chance in hell I was actually going to watch it. I had a lot to learn about my disease but wasn't interested in any of it. I didn't want to acknowledge just how bad it could be, so I focused on the medication that I hoped would make me feel better. All I wanted to do was move on from this whole Crohn's debacle. As if one can "move on" from a chronic illness.

My first prescription was for an iron supplement. Apparently, I was really anemic, which means my red blood cell count was low. My doctor explained that people with Crohn's disease are at risk for anemia caused by a lack of absorption of vitamins and minerals due to inflammation, diarrhea, and blood loss. If the intestines can't absorb enough of the good stuff from the food we eat, the body won't have what it needs to create more red blood cells. Anemia can cause dizziness, coldness, pale skin, weakness, and extreme fatigue, among other things. (Sound familiar?)

No wonder I came home from school every day and slept for hours. No wonder I woke up from sleeping all night only to feel drained and in need of a nap an hour later. No wonder I fell asleep before everyone else at sleepovers. It felt so validating to know I wasn't lazy or out of shape—I was anemic!

The second prescription was for a medication called Asacol that I would need to take for the rest of my life or until it stopped working. Asacol works by decreasing swelling in the colon. In the late '90s, treatment options were limited— so, if the Asacol failed, I could very well find myself in need of surgery to remove the inflamed section of my colon or rectum. The dose was six huge pills three times a day for a total of eighteen jagged little pills: eighteen daily reminders that I was, in fact, sick, different, and broken.

My mom had to constantly remind me to take it because I just couldn't wrap my mind around having to take medication every single day, three times a day, for the rest of my life. I cringed and rolled my eyes every time she asked, "Chris, did you take your medicine today?"

The final prescription was for Prednisone, or as my friend refers to it, "The Devil's Tic Tac." Prednisone is both a miracle drug and a nightmare. The miracle is that within days of taking Prednisone, I felt incredible. I had more energy and could eat without sprinting to the bathroom (more of a fast walk, but still—we were making progress!). And by day six, I had taken my first solid bowel movement in nearly two years. I literally cried tears of joy—no joke. Joy and tears over a solid BM.

Although I felt amazing initially, about two weeks in, the physical and emotional side effects started to kick in. In addition to an increased appetite (I would slam an entire box of cereal in a single sitting), Prednisone can also cause some pretty intense mood swings.

I would experience feelings of euphoria one moment and fits of rage the next. (They don't call it 'roid rage for nothing!) One evening, I had such a surge of energy that I got on our treadmill, listened to *Welcome to the Jungle* by Guns N' Roses on repeat for forty-five minutes straight, and ran my ass off the entire time. Immediately following the G&R-induced jaunt, I verbally attacked my poor mother for kindly asking me if I took my final dose of medicine for the day. I felt like I was losing my mind.

I had never experienced such a rollercoaster of emotions before. I couldn't decipher what was the medicine, what was the shock of my diagnosis, and what was just me. Most days, I felt like I was swirling around inside of a tornado. It was all so confusing. One moment I felt elated and grateful, and the next, I felt agitated and enraged.

Years later, my best friend recalled a time I kicked her out of my car because she apparently pissed me off for who knows what. I told her to get out and walk home, or I was going to "punch her in the face." Note, this is my best friend in the entire world. The person who knows me better than I know myself. The person who would eventually become the godmother to my oldest daughter.

And I was ready to shank a bitch in a steroidal-induced fit of rage.

Prednisone also caused acne, weight gain, and the classic "moon face" associated with steroid use. Looks of pity or disgust replaced the praise I once received for my appearance and thinness. The manager at the pizza shop where I worked flat-out asked me in the middle of a shift, "What's up with your face?" I laughed it off and pretended like I wasn't devastated. Of course, I didn't tell him what was going on with my health. Instead, I swallowed my embarrassment and let it fester in my already fragile gut.

Medication, pamphlets, and videotape aside, you know what no one gave me or my parents? A referral to a therapist to talk through all the big, scary, heavy things I was feeling. How in the world is a seventeen-year-old with such little life experience supposed to process a chronic illness that could impact her ability to live a normal life, have children, and potentially need multiple surgeries, including an ostomy bag? Big miss, Doc. Big miss.

Immediately after my diagnosis appointment, my parents picked up my older brother and baby sister, and we all headed to the mall. Retail therapy was the best they could do at the time.

My mom and I walked around my favorite store. I felt numb as I perused the racks of clothing. *What is going on? Why are we at the goddamn mall right now? Are we just going to pretend this isn't happening?*

"Pick out a new outfit. Anything you want! Something cute. Maybe a new dress will cheer you up." My mom so desperately wanted to make me happy. I can only imagine how helpless she must have felt, not knowing exactly what to say or do for me. She couldn't take away my pain, but she could drown it in new clothes.

I halfheartedly picked out a Gwen Stefani-esque slip dress (think *Tragic Kingdom* circa 1995 ... not the sparkly, glammed-out Gwen of today) and pretended to be jazzed. I had a new dress to go with my new diagnosis.

It felt like a consolation prize. *Tell her what she's won, Vanna! Crohn's disease AND a brand-new dress from Express!* What's strange is that I don't remember the moment my parents actually told my brother and sister about my diagnosis. And I don't recall talking about it beyond comments like "It's going to be okay" and "Look on the bright side, it could be so much worse."

Fuck the bright side! I just got diagnosed with a chronic illness that I barely understand and sure as shit don't want to deal with for the rest of my life!

I realize these types of comments were my parents' way of trying to make me feel better, but all they made me feel was guilt and shame for being anything other than grateful.

When we got home from the mall, I retreated to my bedroom and called a friend I worked with at the local pizza shop. I made the conscious decision not to call my best friend but some guy I had known for less than three months. Calling my best friend felt way too vulnerable, and I didn't want to deal with anyone else's emotions that I loved or loved me.

"So, what's the deal, kid?" He was in college and thought it necessary to speak to me like I was a four-year-old.

"The doctor said I have something called Crohn's disease," I said, feeling as though I was talking about someone else— anyone else—but me.

"Wow, really? My grandfather actually died of complications from that." *Not helpful, dude. So not helpful.*

"Really? Oh ..." I trailed off and carried on the conversation for another fifteen minutes or so, pretending as if what he said didn't terrify me. This is precisely where a therapist would have been a really helpful addition to my plan of care.

It turns out I wasn't the only one trying to process the events of the day. Years later, I found out my parents spent the evening in their own bedroom crying and pacing and bargaining and blaming themselves and each other for my diagnosis. How could this happen? Whose fault was it? And what did it all mean?

For parents, a sick child is a pretty tough pill to swallow too.

"I had a lot to learn about my disease but wasn't interested in any of it."

CHAPTER 5

TRUST ISSUES

———

It's fair to say I have trust issues.

Not so much with other people, but more so with myself—more specifically, with my body. This happened long before my diagnosis, although that certainly didn't help.

As a child, I remember getting a lot of positive attention for my body and overall appearance. Family members would often comment on how "skinny and lanky" my body was as if it were some great talent worthy of praise and admiration.

While the women on my mom's side of the family seemed to be in a perpetual state of dieting, I clearly took after my dad's mom, who would often recount how she only weighed one hundred pounds on her wedding day. Apparently, she hated being so skinny and did everything she could to try and gain weight. As a kid, I remember being confused by the concept of "too skinny." *Did such a thing exist if it came with so much praise?*

When I was a teenager, my mom often told me that total strangers would stop her on the street and comment on what a beautiful child I was—and how uncomfortable it made her. My mom has never been great at taking a compliment, and even as a kid, I could sense her discomfort at these comments. It made me uncomfortable too, but I wasn't exactly sure why.

As I entered my teen years, I started getting attention from men. One evening after babysitting, the dad drove me home and complimented me on my eyes and "shapely legs." I never wore shorts again when I babysat for that family and begged my mom to pick me up so I wouldn't have to be alone in the car with "Captain Creepy Dad." I was fourteen.

Sometimes when I was out with my parents, a guy would make a comment, and my dad would get mad and yell, "She's only fifteen! What the hell is the matter with you?" Of course, I would be mortified and swore up and down I could take care of myself. The reaction from my father, while totally understandable, only added to the discomfort I felt about my body.

To be clear, I never really got it. When I looked in the mirror, I saw an average-looking Italian girl with brown eyes, black hair, and thick eyebrows; who got her upper lip waxed once a month. But after a while, I started to buy into the hype even though that's all it ever felt like to me.

As a freshman, I took geometry with upperclassmen and would overhear the older boys talk about me. At first, it was super flattering. But eventually, they started saying inappropriate things and grabbing my butt when I walked past them. I laughed it off because I didn't know what else to do. But it became so distracting and upsetting that I decided to say something to my teacher even though I was scared.

You would think my teacher would have immediately yanked those little assholes out of the classroom and sent them to the principal's office, or—at the very least —move my desk so I wouldn't be sitting in the lion's den, among all of them. You would think my teacher would want to protect his student and use this as a teachable moment with the boys on how to respectfully speak to and treat a young woman.

You would be wrong. My teacher did none of those things.

"Chrissy, don't you think you bring this attention on yourself?" His response crushed me. I instantly felt the sting of embarrassment and shame. *It must have been my fault this happened. I must have done or worn something wrong. This is all my fault. I shouldn't have said anything.*

I didn't dare tell my parents what was going on at school because I thought I would get in trouble. They often lectured me on the importance of being humble and modest. Yet, whenever we would go anywhere as a family, I was expected to put on a dress and look pretty. As a young girl, it was confusing to be both celebrated *and* punished for something so trivial as my appearance. But, by my sophomore year, the scale seemed to tip toward punishment.

* * *

I got my first job working at a pet store, which was comical because I wasn't exactly an "animal person." I would often gag at the smell of the hamster cages and pig-ear dog chews. But I made an exception and learned to live with the stench because I was so excited to earn my own money. Independence was and has always been very important to me.

The first few weeks on the job were great. I learned how to operate the cash register, process returns, and close down my drawer for the night. I had fun talking with customers and getting to know my older coworkers. Within a few weeks, the assistant store manager started showing me more attention. He asked what I liked to read and complimented me on how mature I was for a fifteen-year-old girl. It all seemed pretty harmless and made me feel special.

But his attention quickly went from harmless to inappropriate. He started calling me sexy, asked to take me to lunch, and offered to drive me home from work after every shift. Each time he offered, I felt sick to my stomach and made up an excuse as to why I couldn't be alone with him.

I mean, receiving compliments from a thirty-year-old man was one thing. Being alone in a car with a thirty-year-old man who thinks it's okay to tell a fifteen-year-old girl she's "sexy" is quite another.

One evening his patience ran out. I was in the back room stocking shelves, and when I turned around, he was standing there watching me. "Jeez, you scared the heck out of me!" I giggled, holding a can of dog food.

Before I could say another word, he pushed me up against the wall and started aggressively kissing me. And I froze. I felt scared and upset. Not at him but at myself. At that moment, I heard my math teacher's words ring in my ears and felt ashamed. *It's my fault this happened.*

Years later, I told my dad what happened. "Why didn't you come to me?" he asked, looking hurt. I shrugged and pretended like it was no big deal. Plus, I was pretty sure my dad would have made a huge scene and murdered the guy. For some reason, I felt the need to protect my dad *and* the assistant manager.

Instead of telling anyone, I just stuffed it down and prayed the guy would leave me alone. Every time we worked together, I felt panicky and self-conscious. I stopped wearing makeup to work, hoping he wouldn't notice me. I figured if I just stayed quiet and small, he'd lose interest. Eventually, he was transferred to another store.

A few months later, I found another part-time job at a clothing store that sold out-of-style Woolrich sweaters and acid-washed Levi's jeans. The owner was an older gentleman who had a reputation for being a little "unusual." Within a few days of working with him, the comments started.

At first, he'd compliment my outfits in general. Then he started calling out the pockets on the backside of my jeans and how "nice they looked" on me. I remember thinking, *Jesus Christ, not again!*

This time around, I knew what to do. I was quiet as a mouse and didn't engage in any more conversation with this man than was necessary. I folded clothes, rang up customers, and cleaned out the dressing rooms. One night he offered to drive me home in his Ferrari. I politely declined and drove home feeling that familiar sickness in the pit of my stomach.

That feeling was desperately trying to tell me something, but at sixteen, I didn't understand what it meant—other than fear and shame. So, I ignored it and told myself I was being overly dramatic. But somewhere deep down, beyond my past experiences and conditioning, I knew better. I knew I wasn't wrong but didn't trust myself or my body because I was never taught how.

One Saturday, I was scheduled to work all day alone with the owner. About halfway through the shift, he approached me with a request. "Go next door and get me an iced tea, a pack of gum, and a newspaper. *Not* the top copy, though!" He threw me a ten-dollar bill and walked to the small office in the back of the store.

I did exactly as I was told (although I strongly considered purchasing the top copy of the newspaper just to stick it to him!). When I returned, he called me from the back of the store.

"Just bring everything here," he barked. I rolled my eyes as I headed to his office. When I walked in, I was stunned to find him sitting in a chair with his pants unzipped and completely opened. I stood there for a moment, unsure of what was actually happening.

He smiled, looked me straight in the eye, and said, "My shirt got stuck in my zipper. I suppose it would be inappropriate to ask you to help me with this?" My stomach dropped, and once again, I froze.

"I ... um ... I think a customer just came in ... um ... I'm going to go help them," I stammered. The owner never came out of his office the rest of the day, and I stayed glued to the register, my heart pounding the entire time.

After my shift, I hurried to my car and instantly burst into tears. I never went back to the store again. My mom asked me why I quit; I mumbled back something about the clothes in the store being "super lame." Again, I didn't tell anyone about the incident until years later, when I realized how insanely wrong all of these experiences were. All I could figure at that time was that it must have been my fault this happened. There is something wrong with *me*.

Between the negative attention I drew from creepy men and the pain caused by my Crohn's, my body started to feel unsafe, and I wanted nothing to do with it. In fact, I became really angry and resentful of my body. How could I trust something that made other people and myself so uncomfortable? How could I trust something that could unpredictably break down or be attacked at a moment's notice?

Here's the problem with that type of thinking: if I couldn't trust my body, by definition, I couldn't trust or really know myself, which is a terrible way for a young girl or woman to live. Because to truly understand and honor ourselves, we must fully feel and inhabit our one precious body and spirit.

I still had a lot to learn—and even more to unlearn.

"If I couldn't trust my body, by definition, I couldn't trust or really know myself."

CHAPTER 6

HIBERNATION

———

November has always been a hard month for me. It could be blamed on the change in weather or daylight savings. Those are certainly contributing factors, but there is a bigger, heavier reason why November always feels like heartache and claustrophobia. It's the month I was diagnosed with Crohn's disease. It's also the month in which—one year later, during my freshman year in college—I had made myself throw up for the first time. For many years after my diagnosis, November represented pain and hiding.

In elementary school, we learn that animals hibernate for the winter; to survive the long, cold months ahead. Then they wake up in the spring all refreshed, hungry, and ready to get on with their lives. They make it through the dark, harsh winter by falling asleep for months at a time. Their system slows down to manage this process. It's nature's way for bears, bats, and butterflies to survive without having to find food or migrate somewhere warmer.

There's a reason why humans don't hibernate. We weren't meant to fall asleep and hide away in a cave from the cold. We are meant to stay present and awake to all of winter's majesty, beauty—and yes, bitterness. Our bodies weren't designed to shut down; they were designed to adjust. They were designed to huddle together, be nourished with warm meals and family gatherings. To be fully conscious and to feel.

For me, Crohn's disease was a dark, cold winter, and bulimia was my failed attempt at hibernation. I wasn't ready or prepared to face the icy winds of change, sadness, and fear that came with my diagnosis. All I wanted to do was hide and pretend it wasn't real.

By my freshman year in college, everyone had moved on with their lives, and I felt like I should too. But there was a heaviness lodged in my throat that wouldn't let me. I watched my friends pack up and move away to college. I watched my parents learn to adjust to having a daughter with a chronic illness. As Robert Frost once said, "In three words I can sum up everything I've learned about life: it goes on." So, I took my cues from everyone else and decided to keep trucking ahead. I swallowed my fear and sadness—and threw myself headfirst into college life.

College felt like a new beginning, and I was ready to prove to everyone just how *fine* I was. But try as I might, I just could not shake the feeling of rage deep within me. Unlike the early months after my diagnosis when anger would bubble over in a fit of steroid-induced psychosis—this was different.

It was internal. It was self-directed. I had made an enemy out of my body and was ready to show her who was boss. *You want to try to slow me down? Fuck all the way off a cliff, Crohn's.*

I immediately threw myself into college life and my studies. I rushed a sorority, got straight As, went to parties, smoked Marlboro Lights, drank cheap White Zin, and danced with smarmy fraternity boys until 3 a.m. On the outside, I had mastered the art of looking fine; but on the inside, I was sinking and doing absolutely nothing to nourish my body or spirit.

Despite being surrounded by new friends, I felt anxious, unsettled, and lonely all of the time. I felt lost and undeserving. I felt disconnected from the truth and unable to process that I was, in fact, grieving. I was terrified of my body and what having a chronic illness meant. I was angry for having to think about things like colonoscopies. I was mortified for having to take suppositories and handfuls of pills every single day. I was frustrated for feeling exhausted all of the time when everyone else around me seemed to have endless amounts of energy. And I was downright pissed that I had to carry all of this alone, while it seemed as though my friends' biggest concerns were which tube top to wear out that weekend.

Decades later, I sat across from a woman who was in my sorority that happened to work at the same company I did. She asked if I kept in touch with anyone from college and started telling me how close she still was with some of our sorority sisters. I confided in her what a wreck I was my freshman year and how I never felt connected to anyone.

"Wow—really? I had no idea!" She was genuinely surprised. "Everyone loved you and thought you were so cool."

"I didn't feel that way at all. I felt like an awkward outsider the entire time," I confessed, feeling the sting of loneliness I felt as an eighteen-year-old girl all these years later.

"I would have never guessed that whatsoever. You seemed to have it all together," she said, "I'm sorry ... I didn't know."

Of course, she didn't know; because, at eighteen, I had become a master of hiding the ugly parts of myself I didn't think anyone wanted to see. The parts of myself I was certain people would run away from if they knew just what a gross disaster I was beneath the cute, bubbly girl I portrayed on the outside. Every day I carried the heaviness of depression, the sharpness of anger, and the buzz of anxiety—and had no idea what to do with any of it. So, I just kept shoving it down and moving forward. And while my new college friends didn't have the foggiest idea, my parents saw me struggling and suggested I see their therapist, Marilyn.

Marilyn was a sweet little grandma-type who my parents saw after my diagnosis to help them learn "healthier ways of communicating" with each other by "validating each other's feelings." My parents fought a lot after my diagnosis and looked to blame each other. As an adult, I can only imagine how devastated they both must have been. As a teenager, I was pissed they were making *my diagnosis* about them.

Although I spent an hour with Marilyn that November afternoon in 1998, I don't remember much of what we discussed—other than me telling her I felt anxious and blaming it on the pressure of college. She explained to me the premise of fight-or-flight and suggested I exercise as a way to manage my stress.

At the time, I had already been struggling with some pretty intense body image issues as a result of returning back to a normal, healthy weight brought on by the Prednisone. And while the suggestion was perfectly valid, in my broken mind, all I heard was her telling me I was fat and needed to work out. And something in me snapped.

When I got home, my mom asked how the session went. I smiled, threw out an insincere "Fine," then locked myself in the bathroom, hung my head over the toilet, and made myself throw up. It was hard at first, but I was determined. I wouldn't let my body fail me again. I was going to win this battle.

Fuck all the way off a cliff, Chrissy.

The first time I made myself throw up, I felt a relief I hadn't since I was diagnosed a year earlier. The lump in my throat temporarily melted, and I felt oddly proud—like I had accomplished something and was finally able to take control of the body that had decided to break down without so much as asking me how I felt about the whole situation. I felt like I found a safe place to dispose of all my sadness, anxiety, and—most importantly—my rage. It felt good to rid myself of all the things I didn't want to feel or face. At least, that's what I told myself.

Once I got a taste of this new hiding place, I dove in head-first. I got addicted to the simultaneous high and emptiness I felt after I would make myself throw up. Anyone who has struggled with addiction knows the feeling of release that comes with erasing oneself with their weapon of choice ... drugs, alcohol, sex, bulimia, work. These are all very dangerous hiding places. But we convince ourselves they're safe because they temporarily take away the feelings we want to avoid at any cost.

The problem with this type of self-destructive hibernation is that it's a soul-sucking, frozen wasteland of shame that only magnifies our pain. It's a lie. A mirage. And it prevents us from doing the real work of healing and grieving.

Let's talk about grief for a moment, shall we? According to *Psychology Today*, grief is "the acute pain that accompanies loss. Because it is a reflection of what we love, it can feel all-encompassing."

There are also phases of grief which most of us learned about in a Psych 101 class; or from someone like Oprah. While there is some debate about the number of phases, the basic gist is this: you have to go through these phases in some form or fashion in order to reach acceptance.

Not around them.

Not underneath or over top of them.

But right smack dab through all those shitty feelings and phases.

There are no shortcuts. You can't run away from or achieve your way out of grief—trust me, I tried. Plus, grief wasn't even on my radar.

At the time, I had a very myopic view of grief. In my mind, it was reserved strictly for the death of a loved one. It wasn't until years later I realized grief applies to the death of anything. A relationship. A dream. A functioning colon. There are so many times that grief is absolutely warranted, but at eighteen, I didn't feel I deserved to grieve and certainly didn't know how.

Everyone around me kept saying things like, "It could be so much worse," or "At least it's not cancer," or my personal favorite: "But you don't look sick." I realize comments like these were meant to make me feel better, but they had the exact opposite effect. They made me feel guilty and ashamed.

So—on behalf of everyone out there battling a visible, or invisible, illness or disability—please never say those words. We don't need our condition minimized in order to feel better. What we need is love, support, and validation that whatever we are feeling is fair and reasonable. Instead of the old *at least it's not cancer* speech, try one of the following:

I am so sorry to hear that. If you're feeling up to it, I'd like to learn more about your diagnosis and how I can best support you.

Ugh—that sucks. I'm curious to know how this is affecting you physically and emotionally. How can I best support you?

Wow—I had no idea. Thank you for sharing something so personal with me. How can I best support you?

Notice a theme here? We need support, validation, and curiosity. We need people to sit with us in the discomfort and ick. Not try to fix us with meal suggestions or "chin up buttercup" platitudes.

I didn't know how to sit in the murky discomfort of grief, especially for something so seemingly intangible as my health and sense of normalcy. I felt like I had lost myself and my future. The vibrant, optimistic girl I once was, seemed to vanish before my eyes—and I so desperately wanted her back.

Years later, my father confessed he observed this change in me immediately. "You were different after your diagnosis. It changed you." Of course, it changed me! But at that time, I thought I had everyone fooled into thinking I was A-OK.

Eventually, I got help for my eating disorder but continued to flirt with various forms of denial and anger for years until there was nowhere left to hide. Just like fear, the ghost of grief would continue to haunt me whether I wanted to admit it or not. And since I refused to acknowledge grief's ghostly presence, it grew bigger in a petri dish of denial.

The denial fed off my pain until it grew so big I felt as if I would burst inside. And if I've learned anything from living with a chronic illness, it's this: You can only lie to yourself for so long before your body responds with some version of "*Oh hell no!*"

"You can only lie to yourself for so long before your body responds with some version of 'Oh hell no!'"

PART 1 JOURNAL PROMPTS:

- In what ways do you trust your body? In what ways do you not trust your body? How can you build trust with your body?
- In what ways do you hide or hibernate when you feel stressed, overwhelmed, or afraid? What would happen if you didn't hide or hibernate?
- How would you describe to another person what it's like living with your chronic illness or condition? What do you wish more people knew?

PART 2

FLYING

CHAPTER 7

TWO SISTERS

There are very few people in my life that can make me laugh like my baby sister, Lauren, could. According to my mom, the moment she put me on the bus to go to kindergarten, she cried and decided she wanted "one more." Lauren was born the summer after I graduated kindergarten.

I adored Lauren as if she were my own real-life baby doll. She made the cutest faces when she laughed. She would grip the side of her crib, bounce up and down, scrunch her nose, and howl with joy. I would do anything to make her laugh just to see that face and probably tickle-tortured her way too much.

We moved a lot as kids, and I often had to share a bedroom (and at one point an actual bed) with Lauren. Sometimes she would wake up in the middle of the night restless and scared. To get her to go back to sleep, I would snuggle her warm little body close to mine, project a Fisher-Price flashlight on the ceiling that changed colors, and tell her stories until she fell back asleep. One night I woke up soaking wet only to discover the perils of sleeping next to a three-year-old. She had peed all over me in the middle of the night. Needless to say, I was not happy and insisted on separate rooms after that incident.

When I was in sixth grade, we moved from Michigan to Ohio. My parents sold the tiny house where Lauren and I once shared a bedroom and moved into another tiny house. Of all the moves, that was the most difficult. We left our community, our best friends, and the bedroom where I would play out all of my Angela Bower fantasies, dance, write, and daydream.

When we moved, Lauren and I shared a room once again. But this time, my mom scored a set of bunk beds from a garage sale in the fancy part of town, so I wouldn't have to worry about getting peed on.

Some nights, Lauren would fuss a little about feeling sad or scared. So, I would jam my arm between the wall and top bunk mattress and hold her hand until she fell asleep and loosened her grip. Years later, we laughed at how both of our arms would practically go numb—but once our hands met, there was no letting go until sleep came.

I would pretend it annoyed me because I was a bratty preteen who missed her best friend and was getting bullied on the reg at her new school. But secretly, I loved feeling her pudgy little hand in mine as a reminder that someone loved me, and as alone as I felt, I would never be alone as long as I had Lauren.

We moved across town when I was in seventh grade into a split level. Lauren and I never shared another room again. At that point, I wanted privacy and wasn't interested in playing house with my baby sister. I was more interested in hanging out with my older brother and his friends, listening to Pearl Jam, and having weekend-long sleepovers with my newfound friends. It was that move that Lauren and I went our separate ways for years as she morphed into a kid who didn't need to hold her big sister's hand to fall asleep, and I morphed into a teenage girl.

While a six-year age gap is nothing now, there was a period of time when six years might as well have been twenty. Once I got to high school, I was constantly on the go with my friends, extracurriculars, and work. When I started to get sick and eventually diagnosed, I wanted nothing to do with anyone, let alone my baby sister.

First of all, I was up to my eyeballs in denial. Secondly, we were just so different. Lauren was a happy-go-lucky tomboy who listened to "MMMBop" and played silly games with her friends. I was a self-absorbed teenager grappling with a new diagnosis who preferred to listen to Fiona Apple and go out with her boyfriend instead. For years it felt like we had very little in common—until the summer after my freshman year in college, when Lauren got really sick while on vacation.

I have very little memory of this vacation because I wasn't there. My sister and mom went to Myrtle Beach with my aunts and cousins—all of whom are roughly the same age as Lauren. I was busy working and saving money for when I moved into an apartment that autumn and didn't want to go, which looking back now is utterly ridiculous. Who passes up a beach vacation at nineteen to *work*? The only thing I can surmise is that I was still very much in hiding mode and wanted nothing to do with my mom, baby sister, or cousins. I had my eye on the prize, which was freedom in the form of a lofted apartment just off campus with two of my sorority sisters.

Recently, Lauren and I were talking about this vacation and her own health issues.

"I had bad stomachaches from time to time when I was a little kid," Lauren remembered. "But it really hit me when we were in Myrtle Beach. I was sick all week and couldn't figure out why I was in so much pain. Everyone thought I was just homesick." The power of denial never ceases to amaze me.

After that vacation, the pain would ebb and flow as Lauren tried hiding her symptoms and became mad when our mom asked her about them. She saw how much pain our mom was still in as a result of my diagnosis and didn't want to make things worse. "It felt like she was very fragile and I didn't want her to cry or be upset." Lauren felt like she had to be strong for our mom and wanted to protect her. "I would get really angry when she asked me how I was feeling because I knew something was wrong."

Within a matter of weeks, Lauren's symptoms quickly progressed: the extreme pain, diarrhea, and fatigue, as well as a fever that lasted an entire week. I remember Lauren suddenly looking very frail and figured she just had the flu, and I went about living my life.

Deep down, we all knew better—especially my mom. She had been here before, a year and a half earlier, with me and knew exactly how to advocate this time around. She took Lauren directly to my pediatric gastroenterologist, and shortly after, Lauren had her very own diagnosis of Crohn's disease.

Looks like we had more in common than I thought.

"I remember Mom getting really serious when she broke the news to me." Lauren didn't want our mom upset, so she said, "It's OK, Mommy. I'll be OK."

You might think this was the moment where Lauren and I reconnected and solidified our sisterly bond. You would be wrong. By the time Lauren received her diagnosis, I had moved out, and she was left alone to process what I still was barely able to acknowledge.

My heart broke hearing Lauren recant her own diagnosis story all these years later, and I was suddenly struck by a sad thought: *I wasn't there for her.*

She was twelve years old and afraid … and I wasn't there for her. How could I have not gone to her or comforted her? What kind of big sister turns away when her baby sister needs her? I had been there for her as a toddler when she was scared. I had been there for her at bedtime when she couldn't fall asleep. But I wasn't there for her when it mattered the most.

I started to get choked up and apologized, "I'm so sorry Lauren. I should have been there for you and I wasn't." But the truth is, at that time in my life, I wasn't there for myself. I didn't know how to process or cope with all the big, scary feelings and thoughts I was having, other than in really unhealthy ways. If I couldn't comfort myself, how in the world was I going to comfort someone else? Comforting Lauren about Crohn's disease meant admitting it was something a person needed comforting about. And I was still very much in the mode of "it's no big deal."

Plus, let's be honest—I was no one to look up to, even at that time. Although I was in therapy for my eating disorder, I still had bad days. And once I moved out, I found new hiding places in the form of older guys, partying, drinking, and smoking. And without my mom constantly badgering me to take my medicine, I pretty much stopped.

It wasn't until a few years after her diagnosis that Lauren and I reconnected and forged a bond that would last the rest of our lives. I remember the exact day it happened; because it was her fourteenth birthday.

Lauren had her friends over and, for the first time, I saw my sister not as some pesky kid but as a teenage girl who was growing up and wanted to talk about things other than Crohn's disease. I was happy to oblige.

"How many boys have you kissed?" Lauren shyly asked. She and her two best friends lined up on my bed, watching me get ready to go out on a date.

"Ha! I have no idea. Why? How many have *you* kissed?" I teased.

"Chrissy! I'm serious!" she jabbed back. Then she looked at me wide-eyed, leaned in, and whispered, "Have you ever had sex?" Her friends giggled in unison and they all turned bright red.

I was twenty years old and felt torn between telling the truth and lying through my teeth. By that time, I had moved back home for the summer, and Lauren and I had almost become buddies as the age gap started to narrow ever so slightly.

I decided to tell her a PG version of the truth:

"Yes, one time." *Lie.*

"And I was in love." *Truth.*

"And out of high school." *Lie.*

"And we used protection." *Truth.*

They all looked at me as if I'd just told them Santa Claus wasn't real. Like they half knew it was true but were still a little shocked to have it confirmed.

"Alright—that's enough questions for now! I need to finish getting ready," I said while digging through my closet, trying to find my Steve Madden platform slides.

"Where are you going?" Lauren asked.

"This guy named Joey is taking me out to Little Italy for a date." I'd met Joey earlier that summer and was instantly smitten.

When Joey arrived, my entire family was over celebrating my sister's birthday. I asked my aunt if she wanted to meet the guy who was taking me out that night. "Nah—what's the point? I'll probably never see him again," she teased. But Lauren wasn't going to miss a chance to check him out. She ran to the front door in a new pair of leopard-print pajamas she got for her birthday to assess the situation. She looked at him and then looked at me and raised her eyebrows up and down—the universal sign for *hubba-hubba*.

Hubba-hubba indeed.

That "guy named Joey" and I were engaged eight weeks later, and Lauren would stand beside me as my maid of honor the following summer.

We've been thick as thieves ever since.

"If I couldn't comfort myself, how in the world was I going to comfort someone else?"

CHAPTER 8

TWO MONTHS

———

The summer I met Joey, I proudly proclaimed to my parents that I wouldn't even think of getting married until I was at least thirty years old—something they loved reminding me about after I ended up getting engaged my junior year in college, a full decade earlier than planned. But here's the thing … you would have married this guy that quickly too.

I met Joey while waitressing at a local Mexican restaurant that made my hair smell like cilantro and onions after every shift.

That same summer, I was in an on-again/off-again relationship with a guy I'll refer to as "College Boyfriend." Who, looking back, never really knew me because I never really let him. College Boyfriend and I started casually dating when my eating disorder started—and suffice it to say, I was in no shape for a relationship of any kind. But this relationship was easy and became another form of hibernating for me. I kept him at arm's length, and he did the same with me, and we were both fine with that. We were opposites in every sense of the word.

In fact, people used to comment all the time about how different College Boyfriend and I were. For some strange reason, I loved it. He was a few years older, way more experienced than I was, obsessed with music and hip-hop culture, didn't believe in God, smoked a pack of cigarettes a day, and wore the same pair of stovepipe jeans the entire time we dated. No joke ... every single day.

I, on the other hand, was naïve, inexperienced, shamelessly loved Dave Matthews Band, got straight As, and went to church every Sunday since I was a child. We were quite the pair, and what I liked most about the relationship was that I knew deep down he could take me or leave me. And hey, I felt the same way about myself at that point, so we were all on the same page.

I wasn't interested in any form of true intimacy or being seen for anything other than a cute, sweet girl who was fun to have around. And for the eighteen-or-so months we were together, I left his apartment practically every time I had to go to the bathroom and held in every single grumbly bit of gas. Which, if you don't have Crohn's, let me tell you—is hard *and* painful. Sometimes I'd pull the old trick of saying I was going to take a shower before bed, proceed to destroy the bathroom, and then take an actual shower to cover my tracks. But geez—how many showers can a girl take in one night?

Dating with IBD is tricky. When do you bring it up? How do you bring it up? What happens if you're spending the night and have to go to the bathroom like three or four times? What happens if you sleep a little too heavy and quite literally shit the bed? What happens if you're on a long road trip—or short drive for that matter—and all of a sudden you feel an attack coming on, and there's not a rest stop or McDonald's in sight?

P.S. If you've never dropped your pants on the side of the road in a total and utter IBD panic in front of a person you're romantically involved with, then you may never have known true humiliation.

And then there is the whole malarkey about women being pretty, neat, and ladylike. Have you ever smelled a Crohn's fart? It's not cute ... it's downright toxic. The question of when and how to bring up my Crohn's with Joey was never really an issue. It was always known and out in the open. This is likely due to the fact that one evening before we went on our first date, I had a little too much to drink and felt compelled to describe, in painstaking detail, a play-by-play account of my most recent colonoscopy in front of a group of relative strangers ... Joey being one of them. Back then, I loved using my Crohn's as a way to disarm people, and I always used humor to deflect. We were all sitting around in my friend's backyard after the bars closed when I opened with something along the lines of, "Have you ever had a camera shoved up your ass? I have!"

Real classy stuff ... but I'm getting ahead of myself.

I will never forget the first time I saw Joey. I fully realize this is going to sound like the world's cheesiest cliché, but it really was love at first sight. It was a warm evening in early summer, and I had been in the middle of a shift at the restaurant. I was at the hostess station rolling silverware when I looked up and saw two guys at table seven (not my table). One of the guys had strawberry blonde hair and a huge smile; the other had jet-black hair and bright blue eyes and was wearing a buffalo plaid flannel shirt and jeans. Buffalo Plaid Guy literally took my breath away. Not only because he looked like an actual movie star, but because there was something else about him I couldn't quite put my finger on—and certainly couldn't take my eyes off of.

The best I can describe is: in that moment, I knew I loved him. Right then and there. Which is totally ridiculous because we hadn't even uttered a single word to each other.

And even though it made absolutely no logical sense, I just *knew.* I felt this pull toward him as if I had known him my entire life and entire lifetimes ago. What struck me most about him, besides the thick row of eyelashes I could see from fifteen feet away, was how he carried himself.

Looking the way he did, he had every right to be cocky, but I could tell he wasn't. There was kindness and quiet confidence that radiated from him, and it fascinated me. He was completely comfortable in his own skin and I could tell he just knew things—and I wanted him to teach me all of them.

"Whoa, who is that at table seven?" I asked my friend and fellow waitress, who was five years older than me.

"Oh, that's Matt and Joey. I graduated high school with them." She joined me in rolling silverware. "They're in town for the summer and then heading to Philly in the fall. Matt got accepted into UPenn and I guess Joe is going with him."

I listened and kept rolling silverware without taking my eyes off table seven.

"We're all grabbing drinks after work tonight if you want to come with," she offered.

Did I want to come with? Of course, I wanted to come with! There was one problem though—I wasn't twenty-one, and they were all going to the bar next door after our shift ended. Do you think that was going to stop me? Absolutely not.

Neither was the fact that I was wearing a neon-pink t-shirt that reeked of salsa, khaki shorts, and tennis shoes. As I mentioned, I'm more of a dress girl, but there was no way I was going to miss an opportunity to meet this guy. So I sprayed on some Bath & Body Works Cucumber Watermelon in an attempt to cover up the fact that I smelled like a walking taco, dug through my purse for the world's most unconvincing fake ID, strolled into the bar, and did whatever I could to get close to Joey. That was the same night I went on a drunken tirade about Crohn's disease and colonoscopies. Years later, he laughs when he recounts the story. "I was sort of confused as to why you were telling such intimate details about your health to total strangers." Joe has often accused me of oversharing.

I asked if it grossed him out.

"No, not really. I just thought it was a little unusual but didn't really give it a second thought." He shrugged with a smile that, to this day, makes me swoon.

A few weeks later, things just sort of naturally fizzled out with College Boyfriend. I began spending more and more time with Joe, his friend, and people from the restaurant. He was honestly like no one I'd ever met before. He carried a book of poetry in his back pocket not because he was a douchebag but because he genuinely loved reading. He wore Levi's 501 jeans in the middle of the summer, listened to Elvis, lived in San Diego for a bit after graduating college, and had a tattoo of a cross on his arm. He clearly loved his friends and family and had a way of making anyone he spoke to feel like they were the only person in the room.

In the beginning, he totally tried to blow me off. "Sure, I thought you were cute, but you were younger than my sister and that just seemed weird. Plus, I knew I was leaving in a few months to go to Philly so I figured, what's the point?"

Then one night, things changed when we were at the same friend's house where I made my colonoscopy confessional. We were listening to music and drinking red wine—which felt very grown-up—and I asked him to take a walk. For some reason, he agreed, and we found ourselves at the edge of the woods underneath a clear sky with a million stars.

We started talking about our lives and what we wanted for our futures. I think it was the first time he realized I wasn't just some young girl but a woman with ideas and passions bubbling beneath the surface. We had our first kiss under that clear, starry sky—and I knew, without a doubt, my first instincts about him were right.

That week we continued to hang out with the larger group, meeting up after my shifts at the restaurant for drinks and having conversations that lasted well into the morning hours. He made me laugh and feel comfortable in a way no man, or friend for that matter, ever had before. Before Joe, even around my closest girlfriends, I always felt a little awkward and out of place. Like, somehow, I just didn't quite belong and couldn't fully relax and be myself. But with Joe, he made me remember who I was before I got angry and lost after my diagnosis. He made me feel like the very best, most authentic version of myself. He didn't expect perfection—he just expected me.

One morning a group of us piled into Matt's truck to get breakfast after a night of drinking, and, without hesitation or hint of embarrassment, Joe farted. "Oops. Must have been one of them California barking spiders," he joked. In the past, I would have been disgusted by a hot guy farting in front of me; but for some reason, when Joe did it, it just made me giggle and love him even more.

After breakfast that morning, he pulled me aside and asked if I wanted to go to Little Italy with him that night. There was a street festival to celebrate the Feast of the Assumption, and there would be incredible food and music. Of course, I wanted to go. "Totally. Who else is going?" I figured it would be the usual group of people we went out with after work.

"Well, I thought it would be nice if it was just you and me," he said, running his fingers through his wavy black hair. My heart nearly exploded in my chest. That was the evening of my little sister's birthday and was hands down the best first date I'd ever been on.

A week later, my grandmother on my mom's side suffered a stroke, and although we hadn't known each other long, Joe offered to drive me to visit her in the hospital an hour away. I was touched that he wanted to be there for me.

Hospitals and illness tend to make people really uncomfortable. They don't like to see the vulnerability and oftentimes don't know what to say or do. Not Joe. He knew exactly what to say and do—which was show up, hold my hand on the drive to the hospital, and introduce himself to my grandmother without a hint of pity or discomfort.

After we left, my grandmother—through a slurred speech from the stroke—said to me, "Chris, he has a nice smile. It reminds me of your grandpa's. Is he Catholic?"

From that day on, Joe and I were inseparable. On the days I didn't work, we'd go to a local park, lay out a blanket, and read. Then we'd go back to his place, listen to Jeff Buckley, and talk all night about his adventures with Matt in Europe or some of the crazy characters he met while living in San Diego.

We sipped cheap red wine, talked about how unexpected all of this was, and wondered how in the world we were going to make a long-distance relationship work. Joe already signed an apartment lease in Philadelphia, and I was starting my junior year of college.

I would come home from a night out with Joe and say to my mom, "I don't know what I'm going to do when he leaves."

She would raise an eyebrow and smile at me slyly, "That boy isn't going anywhere."

By October—a short two months after our first date—Joe asked me to marry him and, of course, I said yes.

"There was something else about him I couldn't quite put my finger on—and certainly couldn't take my eyes off of."

CHAPTER 9

TOO FAST

———

Ever since I was a little girl, the adults in my life have been telling me to slow down.

Slow down—you're going to get hurt!

Slow down—you're eating too fast and going to choke!

Slow down—you're talking too fast. I can't understand a word you're saying!

For the record, I *hate* when people tell me to slow down—even though 99.9 percent of the time they are absolutely correct. I still hate it—almost as much as I hate it when someone tells me to *just relax.*

When I was five years old, my Papa used to take me on walks around the neighborhood. More often than not, he would return furious because I ran ahead. My Nana loved telling this story and got a real kick out of what a little busybody I was and how worked up my Papa would get about the whole situation. "There's no slowing that girl down," he'd say, exasperated.

In September 2015, my last living grandparent—my Nana—had a stroke. The grandmother who had a stroke when Joe and I first met had passed away years earlier. I rushed to the ER straight from work, and my heart broke when I saw her lying in a hospital bed hooked up to machines. I held her hand and asked how she was doing.

She looked up at me with her glassy blue eyes. "I was thinking of you today."

"Me? Why were you thinking of me today?" I said, surprised and assumed she was confused due to the stroke.

"I was thinking about how upset Papa used to get when he would take you on walks." She spoke slowly, her speech slurred. "He would always say, 'If that girl doesn't slow down, I'm not taking her with me on walks anymore!' He would get so nervous because you would run ahead." She smiled and closed her eyes. She really did love that story.

I stood over her and watched her chest slowly rise and fall. I heard the *beep, beep, beep* of the monitors. I saw her struggling to hold on to her smile and felt her hand ever so faintly squeeze mine three times—the universal sign for 'I love you.'

I took a deep breath, looked at my beautiful, patient Nana and lost the ability to exhale. My heart shattered into a million pieces, and it felt like an elephant was sitting on my chest. I immediately ran out of her room and started crying. I let the feelings of fear and sadness creep in and started hyperventilating—like a full-blown, get-me-a-paper-bag-to-breathe-into-I-need-to-sit-down-because-the-room-is-spinning panic attack.

Here was my eighty-year-old grandmother, on arguably one of the worst days of her life, thinking about *me* and my inability to slow down. She knew me well as a child and knew me even better now.

Earlier that day, I was running one thousand miles per hour, preparing for what I perceived as the most important meeting of my career. I was irritable, frustrated with myself, and mentally exhausted from what felt like twelve straight hours of mental and physical sprinting.

I was also ashamed to admit to myself that I hadn't thought about her once that day, that week, and—if I'm being perfectly honest—that month. Oh no, not me. I was much too busy running away from myself to slow down.

In November, my Nana passed away, but not before reminding me how to slow down. I spent the last few months visiting her on weekends and evenings, giving her massages and singing her the same songs she used to sing to me as a child.

* * *

In the summer of 2001, Joe and I married, nine months after our engagement. It was the summer before my senior year in college. We had no savings, no careers, no plans other than to love each other and build a life from the ground up. My parents kept asking us why we were in such a rush and suggested that we wait until I graduated college. I didn't want to hear a word about waiting ... fast was just my natural speed.

By the time I was twenty-four years old, I was charging full steam ahead. In addition to having been diagnosed with a chronic disease, overcoming an eating disorder, getting married, graduating college, and starting my career, Joe and I bought a house (a major fixer-upper) and became parents for the first time to a beautiful—albeit colicky—little girl we named Stella. Most twenty-four-year-olds I knew were living some watered-down version of *Sex in the City*, minus the Manolo Blahnik heels. Or at least that's what it felt like to me. I mean ... I drove a minivan, for Christ's sake.

Looking back, I subconsciously felt like I was on borrowed time because I had a chronic illness and wanted to squeeze every bit of juice out of life as possible. I lived in fear that another flare-up was always just around the corner, waiting to destroy me. I wasn't interested in slowing down. Terrified—I thought that if I did, that scary, rabid dog would catch up with me. So, I just kept going and going and going like the Energizer bunny.

When I was twenty-seven, we had our second daughter, a spirited little girl we named Roma. While my first pregnancy was pretty uneventful, I had a terrible flare-up with Roma that required me to take an eight-week course of Prednisone. Between the hormones from the drugs and hormones from my pregnancy, I was one crabby pregnant lady.

Unfortunately, the Prednisone didn't work as it did in the past, and I continued to flare even after I took my last dose. Having a newborn and a three-year-old is exhausting. But having a newborn, a three-year-old, *and* an active Crohn's flare-up is downright torture.

But did I let that slow me down? Nope! I was back at work within six weeks and started traveling two weeks after that for a new job I got right after I found out I was pregnant. I was afraid of letting down my new boss and even more terrified of the mounting student loan and credit card debt piling up. So, I just kept hustling while inflammation ravaged my body and fear began to deteriorate my spirit.

"I subconsciously felt like I was on borrowed time because I had a chronic illness and wanted to squeeze every bit of juice out of life as possible."

CHAPTER 10

TOO BUSY

———

When Joe was in his early thirties, he decided to train for and run a marathon. He researched the best shoes, the best gadgets, and read practically every book, magazine, and blog on the subject. Personally, I felt like he was overcomplicating the whole thing. He actually wasn't.

In order to run a marathon at a decent pace, there are best practices that can help runners be successful: things like listening to your body, proper hydration, rest, and pacing yourself—the exact things I always had a really hard time incorporating into my everyday life. (This is also probably the reason I've never attempted to run a marathon.)

For the average person, it's practically impossible to run a marathon at a sprint's pace. It's simply not sustainable. The same goes for life, but I sure as hell wanted to try. Not because I was trying to get to a specific destination, but because I was running away from myself. Throughout my twenties, I kept charging full steam ahead, and as many times as I heard people telling me to slow down, I just couldn't. And I was starting to become reckless.

Having Crohn's as a young mom, wife, and professional felt so inconvenient. I wasn't about to let it get in the way of all the things I felt absolutely needed to get done on any given day. Between work, endless emails, laundry, and bedtime routines—listening to my body didn't seem feasible. And making time for my marriage wasn't even on my radar. *Shhhhh—go away, Crohn's! No time to deal with you right now.*

How foolish I was to think that by ignoring my symptoms, they would just magically disappear. Slowly but surely, they grew louder and louder against the backdrop of my hectic life.

During this time, Stella started preschool; and my youngest daughter, Roma, was in that clingy toddler phase where she insisted on being carried at all times. Looking back, I would give anything to hold my girls on my hip one more time. Now that they're teenagers, I'm lucky to get anything more than a quick "side hug" on most days.

But back then, the extreme fatigue and pain from my Crohn's made holding anything other than my own body upright seem practically impossible. My patience was constantly being tested, not because of frustration with my kids but because of frustration with *myself.* And yet, I wasn't willing to take care of myself. I would put anything and everything before my own needs and then be irritated for taking on more than I could handle at work and home.

And because I had become a master of hiding my illness behind a smile and makeup (by this time, I had perfected the fancy airport woman façade), I didn't even look all that sick; or seem to struggle as badly as I actually did. I refused to admit to anyone, myself especially, just how bad things were getting.

With each passing week, it felt like an invisible force was turning up the speed on a treadmill, on which I was sprinting morning, noon, and night. I never set any kind of boundaries in any aspect of my life, especially at work, because I didn't know how. I used to sleep with my Blackberry and respond to work emails in the middle of the night just to prove my dedication. I sacrificed my basic need for a proper night's sleep for a job I hated, working for people who did not have my best interest at heart. Essentially, I was more loyal to them than I was to myself.

By the way, no one was making me do anything. No one was telling me I couldn't take a nap or day off work. No one was telling me I had to answer emails all hours of the day and night. And no one was telling me I had to keep pushing and working and striving. I did it all to myself. I had choices. We always have choices. And I chose not to exercise any of them. Let's be clear ... inaction is a choice too.

* * *

Early on, Joe and I decided we didn't want to put our girls in daycare, so until Stella was in first grade, he was the primary caregiver. Back then, a stay-at-home dad was a relatively new concept and not one a lot of people (i.e., my family) appreciated or understood. Joe also taught English part-time at a community college a few nights a week to help make ends meet.

There were days I would wake up at 4:30 a.m., drive three hours to a meeting, make a few sales calls, and drive all the way home slamming coffee and smoking cigarettes the entire time just to stay awake. Then I would spend the rest of the evening in the bathroom, with the girls, or distracted on my phone trying to catch up on emails. By the end of each day, I was so drained and had very little of myself left to give to anyone—especially Joe.

Between my work schedule, his teaching schedule, and caring for the girls, some pretty thick walls started to form between us, especially regarding my job—which had me traveling all the time, or out in the evenings, entertaining clients. Tension and resentment started to build, and the busier Joe and I got, the less time we made for each other. But it didn't even feel like there was time to spare. My marriage, like my Crohn's, would just have to wait.

Things were slowly starting to fall apart because I refused to admit I was stressed, exhausted, and honestly terrified. But of course, I didn't tell my husband or anyone else for that matter. So, I kept myself busy and pushed Joe, my family, and friends away. I thought if anyone got too close, they would see how bad things were, and I wasn't interested in hearing any of it. So, I hid my pain.

Here's the thing I didn't realize about chronic pain and fatigue. For me personally, it turned me into a real jerk. I could see myself becoming negative, impatient, and angry but didn't know how to stop. The sicker and more exhausted I became, the harder I ran. I literally felt like I was possessed by some awful version of myself. And boy, was I angry.

I was angry with my husband.

I was angry with my friends.

I was angry with my parents.

I was angry with total strangers.

Most of all, I was angry with myself.

My whole life—people used to describe me as an energetic and optimistic person. I wanted to make everyone happy, comfortable, and feel loved. I was a glass-half-full kind of gal who was madly in love with her husband and life. But by the time I was in my late twenties, I had no idea where that girl went. I thought she was gone and figured this stressed-out, reactive, crabby jerk was all that was left.

Of course, that wasn't true. I wasn't actually a jerk. I was sick. And I was terrified to admit I needed help and to learn how to love and take care of myself. I hid the truth from everyone, or so I thought. And little by little, my body started acting out.

At first, she tried whispering to me nicely.

"Pssst. Chris, it's me ... your body. Something isn't quite right, and I need you to see me and take care of me."

I ignored her.

"Um ... hello! Anyone there? I know you see this blood, and I know you feel this constant pain. What's the deal? You gonna help me out here or what?"

Take a number, sister! I've got ninety-nine things to deal with at the moment, and you're not one of them. But, I'll call the doctor next week or whatever. It's fine. You're fine. Now stop pestering me, and let me get back to work!

"You have been putting me off for the past two years and I am not having it anymore. I'm sorry that it's come to this, but I've let you take the lead for far too long. It's my turn now."

My body was sick of my shenanigans and refused to be ignored any longer. On my twenty-ninth birthday, she set into motion a series of events that would ultimately change my life and our relationship with each other. And by the way, my body was right. She needed love and attention, and if I wasn't willing to give it to her, she had every right to fight for it. And boy, did she fight.

2009

On the day of my birthday, my family and I went to my parents' house for a little get-together. We had cake, opened gifts, and I spent the majority of our visit in the bathroom.

At that time, I could still snow my husband with the whole "I'm fine" bit, but my mom knew better.

"Chris, what's going on? You don't look so good. You feeling okay?"

"Ya, I'm fine. Just having an off-day with my Crohn's."

More like an off-year, but who's counting?

"You've been spending a lot of time in the bathroom, and you seem to be in a lot of pain," the woman wasn't about to let me off the hook that easy.

I pushed a piece of cake around on my plate, avoiding eye contact. "I actually have a doctor's appointment tomorrow. I'll adjust my medication and probably start feeling better in no time."

Mothers know when their children aren't well, and she was right. I was in a lot more discomfort than usual. In addition to the cramping, gurgling, and blood, I started getting sudden, sharp pains at the top of my stomach; that radiated around to my back. It felt like somebody was shoving a knife right through the middle of my body. It reminded me a lot of labor pains—in that the sensation took my breath away and progressively grew stronger and sharper throughout the evening.

Eventually, I retreated to the couch and curled up under a blanket with a heating pad for an hour before I finally conceded. The pain wasn't going away. If anything, it was getting stronger. "Hey, Mom," I shouted from the couch while she was cleaning up after dinner.

"I think something is wrong." My voice cracked from another wave of pain. I felt as though I might actually pass out. "Do you mind if the kids stay here tonight so Joe can take me to the ER?" I tried my best to sound unaffected and casual, as if I were asking her to babysit, so Joe and I could go out on a date.

She stopped her cleaning frenzy and looked at me as if I were insane. "Yes, of course! Please go and please take care of yourself. Chris, you need to slow down."

And there they were ... the two words I hated most.

I could tell how worried she was, and for some reason, it annoyed me. Mostly because I also felt worried and because she made the concept of slowing down seem so easy. As if slowing down was even an option at that point in life. (Spoiler alert: It's *always* an option. I just didn't know it applied to me.)

* * *

I get quiet when I'm in pain or scared, and since we were batting two for two in that moment, the drive to the hospital was relatively silent. Joe drove with one hand on the wheel and one hand on my arm. I could tell he was starting to worry, which also annoyed me. I briefly winced as a wave of stabbing pain returned. I tried to downplay it, but he could tell because my whole body tensed.

"Oh, babe. It's okay. We're almost there," he said gently.

I smiled at him as a way to prove things weren't that bad. "No worries." I waved my hand. "Remember I've had two babies and have been through a lot more pain than this!"

It was a quiet Sunday evening at the hospital—and, as a result, I was able to get checked in immediately. A nurse started an IV with some medication to lessen the pain, took my blood, and collected a urine sample. After a few hours, we had an answer.

The doctor walked in with a clipboard and cheery demeanor. "Okay, I think we found the problem." He scratched his head with the tip of his pen. "Your bloodwork shows your amylase levels are elevated. That, paired with the placement of your pain, suggests pancreatitis."

"Oh, okay. What does that mean? Do I need antibiotics?" It was after midnight by that time, and I yawned, assuming it was similar in severity to a urinary tract infection.

He suggested I should probably check in to the hospital for a few days until things settled down. That snapped me awake! I was shocked by his suggestion. What in the world was this man talking about? A *hospital stay?* My negotiation skills kicked in as I flashed him a smile. "Is that really necessary? I actually have an appointment with my gastro tomorrow, and I really don't want to miss it because it takes so long to get in with him."

The doctor paused for a moment and scratched his head one more time before responding. "Okay. Take this paperwork with you when you see your gastro tomorrow. Let him know you were here tonight and the diagnosis. I'll write you a prescription for medicine to manage the pain, but you really need to take it easy the next week or so. Lots of rest, lots of liquids, bland food, and no alcohol."

Deal! I grabbed the paperwork, signed out, and we headed home.

The following morning, I arrived at my doctor's appointment bright-eyed and bushy-tailed, as if I hadn't just been in the ER a mere eight hours earlier. The nurse weighed me, took my temperature, and showed me to my room. It was just like every other exam room I've been in since I was diagnosed twelve years earlier: bland and cold—with cheesy artwork next to posters of a healthy colon and an unhealthy colon. I stared at the posters as I waited for my doctor to come in, wondering what part of my colon was unhealthy this time around.

After about twenty minutes, my doctor walked in and got right down to brass tacks. "Hello, my dear. What brings you in today?"

I smiled and instantly felt the need to be charming in order to make my doctor feel comfortable. I wanted him to like me and think I was a good patient. I told him I was feeling a little symptomatic lately. Which was the understatement of the year.

My doctor opened his laptop and began typing. "What kind of symptoms?"

"The usual ... pain, frequency, urgency." *And fatigue. And blood. And bloating. And a loss of appetite. And extreme irritation with anyone who looks at me sideways.*

"Uh-huh, uh-huh." He typed without looking up. "When you say frequency, how many bowel movements are you having a day?"

"Well, ... it's hard to say ..."

"On average?"

"It depends what I eat but, ... if I had to guess, I'd say about ten or so times a day." *More like twenty, but who's counting?*

"And what is the consistency?"

"Loose. Watery." I began fidgeting with my Blackberry to avoid eye contact. I knew what he was going to ask me next.

"Any blood?"

I paused. I hated to admit there was—because I knew that meant things were bad. Blood is not good. Red means danger. Red means stop.

"Any blood?" he asked again, looking up from his laptop.

"Ya, ... I guess. But not all the time." I smiled, trying to downplay the fact that there had been blood when I went to the bathroom almost every day for an entire year.

He took a deep breath. I could tell he was not happy. "Okay, let me feel your tummy." With ice-cold hands, he pressed on, and around, my abdomen. "Any pain here?" I shook my head no. "What about here?" I shook my head no again.

Here's the thing about pain: it's relative. And after being in pain for more than a decade, it was hard for me to distinguish serious pain from the ongoing discomfort of daily life. Sure, it hurt when he pressed on my abdomen, but not as bad as it hurt any other time.

"What about here?" he pressed on my pancreas, and I let out a small moan.

"Oh yes, I meant to tell you," I said casually—as if I had just remembered to invite him to a dinner party, "I was in the ER last night. Apparently, I have pancreatitis."

"Wait, what? No. You don't have pancreatitis. If you had pancreatitis, you would have been admitted to the hospital." He looked me right in the eyes. "Pancreatitis is really serious."

I handed him my discharge papers from the hospital. He sighed as he looked them over.

Oh man, I was busted. "Is it that bad?" Maybe he wouldn't get mad at me if I played dumb.

"Is it bad? Well, it's not good. Pancreatitis is very serious and, if not properly treated, can kill you." The tone of his voice made me uncomfortable. It was stern and direct. My stomach started hurting even more because I knew he was upset, and I hated feeling someone else's disappointment.

"I just can't believe he agreed to let you leave."

"Well, I can be pretty persuasive." I smiled, trying to lighten the mood. He was not amused.

After some back-and-forth negotiations, my doctor also agreed to let me leave on one condition. I had to promise to head home immediately, stay in bed for the rest of the week, and stick to a clear liquid diet. "Between your colon and your pancreas, you have a lot of inflammation going on, and we need to get things to calm down."

He reopened his laptop and started feverishly typing. "Here's what we're going to do," he clicked away while speaking out loud. He agreed to treat me with a course of Prednisone and rambled on about other medications, including suppositories and Protofoam. If you're not familiar with Protofoam, allow me to enlighten you. Protofoam is a foam you insert into your rectum to help reduce inflammation. Picture inserting a can of Cheez Whiz up your butt, and you'll get the picture. Real charming stuff.

"I want to see you back in my office in two weeks to see how things are progressing. My dear, you need to take this seriously. We need to get this inflammation under control before things get any worse. Do you understand?" His tone was serious and fatherly. I felt like I was in trouble and didn't like being talked to like I was a child—even though I was 100 percent acting like one.

I left his office that morning, picked up my prescriptions, and really did have every intention of following his orders. Then life got in the way. I managed to stay in bed the rest of the day but was back at it Tuesday morning. It started with a few emails and a couple of returned phone calls, then a load of laundry and a quick trip to the grocery store.

Before the week ended, all the promises I made to my doctor and myself went out the window, and I was back on the treadmill of my busy life. My body would just have to wait. She would just have to adjust and figure things out on her own.

I also convinced myself I didn't need to follow up with my doctor two weeks later. I justified this absurd lie by telling myself things like, *There's nothing he can do anyways. It's not like I have a sore throat, and he can look inside me and see what's wrong.* And the ultimate lie: *This is just the way my body is, and it will eventually get better.*

A year later, I read a quote that would forever stay with me. I think of it often when I feel myself slipping into the seductive lure of avoidance. Please, if you have a chronic illness or condition of any kind, remember these words. Repeat them to yourself when you start to get stubborn with your body and life. Tattoo them to your forehead if you must. Drumroll, please ...

Nothing changes if nothing changes.

Take a breath. It bears repeating.

Nothing changes if nothing changes.

One more time for the folks in the cheap seats:

NOTHING. CHANGES. IF. NOTHING. CHANGES.

Period. End of sentence. It's a pretty basic concept I didn't fully realize or understand at that time in my life. I was still very much on the struggle bus driven by fear disguised as a cute, zippy sports car. How in the world did I expect to start feeling better if I wasn't willing to change my lifestyle, listen to my doctor, and, most importantly, my body? How in the world was I going to stop feeling resentment, anger, and anxiety over my disease if I wasn't willing to seek counseling or support?

I was a twenty-nine-year-old mother of two and literally had no idea how to care for myself in the way I needed and deserved—until the infamous black-dress-diarrhea-river-down-my-leg incident that occurred later that summer.

"Let's be clear ... inaction is a choice too."

CHAPTER 11

TOO LATE

———

By July of 2009, my marriage, job, and body went from bad to worse. Joe and I were fighting all the time, the pressure with my job intensified, and I had another bout of pancreatitis that landed me in the ER. By midsummer, I could barely drink a sip of water without getting sick, let alone eat a proper meal. I was going to the bathroom more times a day than I could actually count. Little did I know, I was in for a major wake-up call—involving my favorite black dress, an empty McDonald's bag, and a truly humbling moment in a Hilton parking lot.

On the Fourth of July, we visited my best friend, and she could tell I wasn't in a good place. "Dude, what is up with you?" she asked when we were setting up a movie for our kids to watch before bedtime.

"What do you mean?" I replied, laying out blankets and juice boxes for the girls.

"You're being really mean to Joey and just seem super annoyed." She called me out in a way only a best friend can, and boy, did it irk me. For the record, she was 100 percent right. I was being really snippy with Joe and was super annoyed with everyone. Chronic pain, dehydration, and malnourishment will do that to a person.

"You have no idea what I'm dealing with right now," I snapped back, "I love you, but mind your own business."

I turned away from my best friend and felt a sharp lump form in my throat. I was pissed. How dare she call me out like that! She had no idea the pressure of my job, the tension in my marriage, or the utter exhaustion I carried around with me morning, noon, and night.

When you get to a point in life when you're pissed off at the people who love you the most, chances are you're not living an authentic, wholehearted life. Not even close. What you are living in is fear. And my fear was slowly destroying me from the inside out because I kept slamming down every negative emotion like shots of tequila.

I was drunk on my own ego, and the years of sadness, hibernation, and running that had turned me into a woman I hardly recognized. The girl Joe met at the Mexican restaurant was stone-cold passed out, and this angry, fear-drunken woman had taken over.

The next night after the girls' bedtime routine of baths, jammies, and books, I snuggled both Stella and Roma close to me in bed. These girls were everything—magical little wonders whom I loved so much it hurt. Roma was a little spitfire with big, baby-doll eyes and fluffy cotton-candy hair. Stella was a quiet and bright twinkly star who was simultaneously silly and wise beyond her years. I looked at their sweet little faces, watched their bellies rise and fall as they drifted off to sleep with their favorite blankets, and felt the lump in my throat grow a little bigger.

I felt so much guilt for being tired all the time. I felt shame for being impatient with them when they asked to be picked up. But most of all, I felt afraid. Things were spiraling out of control, and I wasn't doing myself any favors. If they were sick or in pain, I would move heaven and earth to make them feel better and whole. Why wasn't I willing to do the same for myself?

The following morning, I called my doctor to let him know the medication I was taking wasn't working and asked for another course of Prednisone. He was quiet on the other line—so much so that I thought we got disconnected.

"Christine, this has been going on for months. You were supposed to get bloodwork and have a follow-up appointment months ago, and you never did either of those things. And I see here you were back in the hospital with pancreatitis." He sounded so disappointed it pained me.

"I know, I know. I'm sorry. I've been really busy lately, and it just slipped my mind," I bumbled.

"I'm not calling in any more medication until I see you in my office. I had a cancellation this afternoon and can get you in today."

Ugh! I don't have time for that! My temporary bout of vulnerability was replaced with irritation.

"I'm going out of town for work today and won't be back until tomorrow." I had scored a meeting with a very important prospect that took me months to schedule. I wasn't about to miss it. He and my body would just have to wait a little longer.

Silence on the other end. I could tell how annoyed he was, and rightly so. If I wasn't willing to prioritize my health, why should he? There were plenty of other people on his waiting list who were very sick and would do anything to get an appointment with him.

"How about Friday then? That's my last open appointment for weeks. I want to perform a sigmoidoscopy and see what is going on." A sigmoid is like an express version of a colonoscopy. It didn't require the same level of prep as a colonoscopy because it only examined the rectum and lower half of the colon.

"Okay, I'll take it," I conceded.

After I hung up the phone, I hopped in the shower and noticed for the first time how thin I was getting. My hip bones were starting to jut out, and my breasts were basically nonexistent. When I washed my hair, handfuls of it came out and collected at the base of the drain.

When I got out of the shower, I wrapped myself in a towel and saw a grayish ghost of a woman with sunken eyes staring back at me. It was like I hadn't looked at myself, really looked at myself, in a long time. I took a deep breath. The simple act of showering made me feel like I needed a nap. I looked at my bed out of the corner of my eye and fantasized about crawling back in for the next week. I turned to the mirror and started doing what I did best: putting myself back together.

I used two different types of concealer to cover up the dark circles under my eyes. I swiped bronzer, blush, and a little more bronzer onto my cheeks to add color back to my face. I blow-dried my hair, curled it, and put on my favorite black dress. I transformed into the fancy-airport-woman version of myself everyone knew and loved. It was all so simple and superficial, how easy it was for me to trick people into thinking I was fine and completely healthy.

My meeting was two hours away, and although I was careful not to eat or drink too much before I got on the road, I still had to stop three times to use the restroom: once before I even got to the freeway, once at a random gas station next to an Adult Mart in the middle of a cornfield, and once at a trusty old McDonald's, before getting into town.

McDonald's is where I made my fatal error. While I was washing my hands in the restroom, my stomach started growling. I was starving, and the smell of french fries was too strong for me to resist. I foolishly ordered a small fry and Diet Coke and told myself I would only eat a few and very, very slowly, so as not to upset the beast ... my Crohn's. Of all the things I could have eaten, fried potatoes and fizzy, artificially sweetened soda were the absolute worst choices. At that point, I was just so hungry and so tired I'd convinced myself that the fries wouldn't be *that bad*, and the caffeine from the soda would give me the pep I needed to keep going. *Just keep going.*

Within a few minutes, my body responded, and she was not happy.

What the actual hell?

I was a few blocks from my hotel when the grumblings and gurgling started to kick in.

Are you seriously going to put that garbage in me and not expect to pay the price? How many trips to the bathroom and ER is it going to take for me to finally get through to you?

Oh, man. I had really done it now. She was NOT having it. Enough was enough. She tried being nice. She tried being mean. The only tool left in my body's toolbox was pure and utter humiliation.

I pulled off the freeway to check into the hotel I would be staying at overnight. I could see the Hilton Garden Inn two traffic lights away. I started breaking out in a cold sweat from needing to go to the bathroom like, NOW, and the fear that I might not actually make it to the hotel.

I bombed through the first traffic light effortlessly (thank you, Crohn's gods) but got stuck at the second light—not one, but TWO back-to-back red lights because there was so much traffic. By the time the light finally turned green, I knew I was in trouble. I gunned it into the parking lot and whipped my car into the first spot I could find. I had made it! Thank God! I turned off the car, unbuckled my seatbelt, and got out of the car. The moment I stood up was when it happened. I was too late.

In the middle of broad daylight, in my favorite black dress—I shit myself. I stood there for a full minute in total and complete shock. *No way I just shit myself. No freaking way.* I panicked and dug around in my car for something to clean up with—and didn't have so much as a tissue with me. Damn it!

What I did have was a river of diarrhea running down my legs and an empty McDonald's bag, which I crumpled up like toilet paper and attempted to wipe off my legs. (Note: paper bags have zero absorbency.).

You should know this wasn't a proud moment for me. I strongly considered leaving this detail out of the book—but then I would not be doing myself, or the millions of women and men with IBD, any justice. Shitting oneself is par for the course when you have Crohn's or Ulcerative Colitis. And I share the intimate, graphic details of this story with you for a few reasons:

1. For the love of God, be prepared.
2. This is the truth, the whole truth, and nothing but the truth.
3. To illustrate what a hot mess express I allowed myself to become by ignoring my symptoms for so long that it finally took this incident to wake me the hell up.

I checked into the hotel and immediately headed to my room for a shower. While I was in the shower, I leaned against the tile and felt dizzy, drained, and empty. I'd hit some kind of wall and knew I was toast. There was no way I was going to make my dinner that night. I got out of the shower for the second time that day and laid on the bed still wrapped in a towel and soaking wet. The thought of even moving to put on clothes seemed impossible. I grabbed my phone to call and cancel my meeting—the one I was so certain I *had* to attend—and saw that my aunt had texted me:

"Grandma went into hospice today."

This was the same grandma who had a stroke the week after Joe and I had our first date back in 2000. She never fully recovered and had lived in a nursing home ever since. The past year, her health had taken a turn for the worse.

I immediately called my grandma to check in on her. I couldn't imagine how scared and sad she must have felt, and I hated that I wasn't sitting next to her, holding her hand.

"Hey Grandma, it's Chris. Just calling to check in and say I love you."

"Well, hello there!" Her speech was still slurred from the stroke. "How are you, my dear? It's so good to hear your voice."

I told her I heard the news about hospice and how sorry I was, how much I loved her, and how I would be visiting her soon.

"How are you feeling? You know, I was praying for you today. I pray for you, Joe, and the girls every day," she said.

"Well, I need all the prayers I can get. I'm really sick." I finally said out loud what I wasn't able to admit to myself or anyone else for a long time. "I'm just so sick and tired of feeling so sick and tired all the time."

"You know what I pray for you the most, Chris?" She paused as if waiting for me to answer. "I pray for you to slow down."

And there it was. Those famous two words had followed me around my entire life.

"You are always on the go. Always so busy. When are you going to slow down and start taking care of yourself? If you're not going to do it for yourself, do it for me." My grandmother was classically trained in the art of Catholic guilt.

Laying in that hotel bed, alone—I started to cry. She was right. It was time to surrender. "Okay, Grandma," I said, "I'll do it for both of us."

The following morning, I went to see my doctor for what I thought would be a quick sigmoid; and ended up spending the next six days in the hospital—learning firsthand how to slow down the hard way.

"When you get to a point in life when you're pissed off at the people who love you the most, chances are you're not living an authentic, wholehearted life."

PART 2 JOURNAL PROMPTS:

- How has/does your chronic illness or condition impact your physical, mental, and emotional health?
- Fill in the blank:
    - When I'm having a bad day, I feel (blank) about my illness/condition because (blank).
    - When I'm having a good day, I feel (blank) about my illness/condition because (blank).

PART 3

FIGHTING

CHAPTER 12

BRICK WALLS

———

I arrived at the hospital on a Friday morning for what I thought would be a quick outpatient sigmoidoscopy. I figured the nurse would wheel me back to the procedure room, start my drip of Versed, I'd nod off to la-la land, wake up a little groggy, find out I had a smidgen of inflammation, and be sent home with a fresh, new prescription. Easy peasy lemon squeezy.

That's not exactly how things went down.

When I woke up in my Versed-induced state, there were two men standing over my bedside. I yawned and slowly blinked in an effort to make my sleepy eyes focus. One man was stroking my head and saying my name; the other was scribbling something down on a notepad. It took me one more round of yawns and blinks before I realized the two men were Joe and my doctor.

"Oh, hi guys," I said, casually; as if we all just sat down for a nice family meal. I gave a woozy smile—evidence of the sedative's lingering effects. "Everything go okay?"

My doctor shook his head while I tried to stay awake. The drugs made my body feel heavy and warm. For the first time in over a year, nothing hurt, and I felt relaxed. I could see how people could get addicted to that shit.

According to my doctor, the sigmoidoscopy—which examines the rectum and lower part of the large intestines—showed an "alarming amount of inflammation." The plan was to admit me to the hospital for one, maybe two days, to receive a few rounds of intravenous steroids in order to get things to calm down.

Maybe it was the drugs, or maybe I was just so tired of running away from myself, but I didn't even try to put up a fight or negotiate my way out of being admitted. For the first time since I was diagnosed, I actually surrendered.

* * *

Prior to spending what would end up being nearly a week in the Digestive Health Unit of the Cleveland Clinic, I used to think hospitals were a place people went when they were hurt or sick that would make everything better—the grown-up equivalent of mom kissing a boo-boo.

Need a few stitches? Hospital.

Need your gallbladder out? Hospital.

Need a quick peek inside my rectum and colon? Hospital.

I naively thought there was this unspoken code between a patient and a hospital.

I play your little game, and, in exchange, you patch me up good as new and send me on my way until next time.

My hospital stay didn't exactly work that way. And for that, as strange as it may sound, I am eternally grateful. My hospital stay was more of a wake-up call or episode of *Scared Straight* than a tender exchange between mother and child.

Up to that point in my life, I never viewed the hospital as a place of learning and undoing—of breaking down walls and surrendering. But for me, that's exactly what my unexpected stay turned into.

When I walked in for my outpatient procedure that warm July morning, I was arrogant, afraid, angry, and emotionally incompetent. When I walked out (well, "wheeled out" is more apt), I was humbled, vulnerable, and awake in a way I had never been before in my adult life.

The irony is that I left the hospital no better physically than when I arrived. I was still in pain, exhausted, and unable to eat without getting sick, and there was still the same amount of blood when I went to the bathroom. While the hospital didn't magically put my flare-up into remission like I thought it would, it actually did me one better. It put me on a path of real, true healing in a way I never thought I needed. But I'm getting ahead of myself....

* * *

As a teenager, I used to come home every day after school, pop on *The Oprah Winfrey Show,* and be inspired by all the ways in which I, too, could live my best life. I met some of my favorite writers and spiritual teachers, including Iyanla Vanzant, Marianne Williamson, and Eckhart Tolle. To this day, one of my all-time favorite shows and podcasts is *Super Soul Sunday.* Don't even get me started on *Master Class* or *O, The Oprah Winfrey Magazine.* The insight, wisdom, and famous "a-ha moments" always have me shaking my head and saying "a-ha" too.

In one episode of *Master Class,* Oprah talked about instinct, knowing oneself, and listening to the wisdom of the Universe, God, The Divine ... whatever you want to call Her.

"I say the Universe speaks to us, always, first in whispers. And if you don't pay attention to the whisper, it gets louder and louder and louder. I say it's like getting thumped upside the head. If you don't pay attention to that, it's like getting a brick upside your head. You don't pay attention to that—the brick wall falls down." Oprah knows.

Clearly, I wasn't paying attention to any of the whispers. The brick upside my head knocked just enough sense into me to call my doctor and agree to the sigmoid. But by the time I was admitted to my room, the sedatives had worn off, and denial kicked back in. It looked like this was going to be a brick-wall-crumbling type of situation.

Oh man, this was a mistake. My doctor and Joe totally duped me! They waited until I was drugged out and pulled this garbage on me. What a scam! This all seems rather dramatic and unnecessary. And this hospital gown—really? Hospital gowns are for sick people, and I am NOT that sick—surely not sick enough to be here. I'm not like the rest of the people on this floor. I am fine. Just a little flare-up, like all of the other little flare-ups I've had before.

The self-gaslighting was truly magnificent.

Whatever. I guess since I'm stuck here for the next two days, I might as well get a little rest and try to relax. I mean, I am exhausted, and if the medicine can just do its thing, maybe they'll let me out a little early!

The delusions were quite grand.

So, I rolled my eyes, hunkered down in bed, popped on the TV, and looked around my room—which felt more like a prison cell. To my left was a curtain that divided the room, and I prayed it would stay that way. I wasn't here to make friends or idle chit-chat with my roommate. This wasn't summer camp! To my right were beeping machines and an IV pole with a bag of clear liquid hanging from the top and a long plastic tube that pumped medicine and saline into my body. Within five minutes, I was already restless. And hungry. I hadn't eaten since the evening prior, and it was now nearly dinner time. I buzzed the nurse's station.

"Hi, it's Christine Rich in room 103," I said in my most pleasant voice, "I was wondering if I might be able to order something to eat?" The nurse put me on hold while I imagined warm, saltless mashed potatoes and chicken fingers with honey mustard.

I might even get a little crazy and order chocolate pudding for dessert. Maybe this wouldn't be all that bad. I could get used to a few days of other people doing all the things instead of me. I'll just chill with some daytime television, have a few snacks, get my medicine like a good patient, and be home by Monday morning.

"I'm sorry, Miss. No can do. Says here you're NBM."

What the heck is NBM?

"Nothing by mouth," she said as if reading my mind.

"Wait, what do you mean?" I was genuinely confused.

"Miss, due to your current condition your doctor has ordered gastrointestinal rest. That means you may only have clear liquids. The cafeteria can bring you some chicken broth if you'd like."

OK, ... first the ridiculous hospital gown, and now this? What the actual hell is going on? Am I getting punked? Where is Ashton Kutcher? This is horse shit.

"Wow, OK ..." I trailed off. "Is that really necessary?" I could feel my negotiation skills flaring up, "Maybe some mashed potatoes or a few crackers would be OK?"

The sweetness in her voice turned curt. "Absolutely not. You can have broth, coffee or tea, popsicles, and ice chips."

Cool. Thanks, Nurse Ratched. A meal of ice chips and broth sounds delectable. Forty-eight hours earlier I was about to have dinner at Morton's Steakhouse, but you know what ... this NBM thing sounds way better.

I went from annoyed to downright pissed. Take away a type A girl's laptop, cell phone, food, and family and pump her full of steroids—then you've pretty much got yourself a brick-wall-falling-down situation in the making. Less than twenty-four hours later, that's exactly where I found myself: under a pile of bricks from a wall I engineered and built, brick by stubborn brick, all by myself.

And although I never felt lonelier, I was never really alone. Nurses were constantly coming in and out of my room morning, noon, and night to take my temperature, check my blood sugar, and ask how I felt. "Are you in any pain, dear?" a nurse would gently ask.

"Yes. Yes, I'm in pain!" I barked. "I am starving!"

The nurse offered me a popsicle. "Would you like orange or grape-flavored?"

Hamburger flavored. I want a hamburger-flavored goddamn popsicle with a side of fries! "Grape is fine."

By Monday morning, I lost five pounds, and, despite receiving almost three days' worth of steroids intravenously, my symptoms were still terrible. Although I was living off clear liquids, I was still running to the tiny hospital bathroom every time I so much as took a sip of water. Oh, and to add insult to injury, I had to relieve myself in what's called a "hat" that would collect my waste so the doctors could monitor exactly what was going on. Damn, these nurses and doctors were good. They weren't going to take my word for it. They were going to let my BMs speak for themselves.

"So, what's the plan, doc? What time should I tell my husband to come pick me up?" I was eager to get home, see my girls, and get on with my life.

"Mrs. Rich, I am recommending we keep you for a few more days. You need more steroids and gastrointestinal rest. From what we can tell, your symptoms are not getting better, and there is still an alarming amount of blood in your stool." *Damn poop hat! Throwing me right under the bus.*

"Wait, what? No. You said I would only be here for two days and then I could go home. There must be some kind of mistake. Can't I just go home and take medicine there?" I could feel my heart start to beat faster.

"Absolutely not. You will stay here for another four days ... six days is the maximum number of days we can treat you with steroids intravenously." The bricks were flying at my head fast and furious now. I felt trapped—like a caged animal—and all I wanted to do was run.

My doctor went on to explain that I would be getting a CT scan the following morning and a full colonoscopy sometime after that. I couldn't make sense of what this man was telling me. Didn't he know I had a life to get back to? Didn't he know I'd never spent more than a couple of nights away from my girls, and another four would be unbearable? Didn't he know that laying in this freaking hospital bed, with nothing but my thoughts and feelings, was killing me? Didn't he know that by staying another four days, I was basically admitting defeat and letting the Crohn's win? How the hell was I supposed to run away and hide from all the things I didn't want to know or see about this illness if I was forced to sit in this nasty hospital a minute longer? I swallowed a huge lump in my throat—the biggest one yet—and grunted some version of, "Fine, whatever."

I was far from fine.

And whatever game I had been playing for the past decade was clearly over.

This was worse than I thought.

"*I was humbled, vulnerable, and awake in a way I had never been before in my adult life.*"

CHAPTER 13

ONE SIP AT A TIME

———

It was becoming clear that I couldn't speed my way through this hospital stay, no matter how badly I wanted to. It would be part of my unlearning, and I absolutely hated it.

I laid in my hospital bed sulking like a child when a nurse came in to suggest I take a walk to lift my spirits. She showed me how to unhook myself from the IV pole I was tethered to morning, noon, and night. It was strange—after only three days, the IV pole felt like an extension of my body. It also served as a physical reminder to slow down. Doing something as simple as getting up to use the restroom required me to pause, untangle the tubes, and gently maneuver my body. I had no choice but to move slowly.

"You've got about thirty minutes before we need to hook you back up. I just thought you might want a little break for now." She smiled at me, and for the first time since I arrived, I began to feel something other than anger and fear. I felt a connection.

Prior to that moment, I turned every medical professional into an enemy because the power and control shifted to them. But that afternoon, in that small exchange with my nurse, I started to see the staff for who they really were: dedicated professionals who wanted to see me—a total stranger—get better. They were all working so diligently to do their part. As I took the first step outside my room in three days, I realized it was time for me to start doing mine.

But how?

I walked one very slow lap around the unit, thinking about what was happening, how I ended up there, and what would happen once I left. Would life go back to normal? What even was normal at this point? The tension in my marriage? The stress and demands of my job? The total and utter lack of self-care that made me feel like a walking zombie most days?

As I pondered what changes I needed to make, I saw a young man with a walker coming toward me.

Avoid eye contact. Remember, Chris, we aren't here to make friends.

"Hey there." The boy smiled. "Feel like some company?"

Uuuuugggghhh. Hell no.

"Sure," I mumbled.

It's a weird experience meeting someone for the first time in a hospital. First of all, when is the last time you met someone while wearing a paper-thin hospital gown that ties in the back without a bra on? I met new people all the time for my job at networking events. But then I was prepared, put together, and ready to extend my most confident handshake and megawatt smile. All of that seemed so ridiculous now.

"Hi, I'm David."

"Hey, I'm Christine." I was suddenly aware that I hadn't showered since I was admitted and felt a little self-conscious.

David didn't seem to notice or care. "What are you in for? Is this your first time?"

I must have had "newbie" written all over me. I could feel my wall starting to go up and was irritated by how confidently

David strolled around the unit—giving head nods to fellow patients and saying hello to the nurses by name when they passed us. Who was he ... the goddamn mayor of the Cleveland Clinic? Showoff!

"I came in a few days ago for what I thought was going to be a quick stay for intravenous steroids. Somehow they roped me into staying for six." I could feel David watching me as I spoke, and for the first time, I allowed myself to make eye contact with him. David's face was puffy, and his body was frail. His skin was the color of bland oatmeal. He didn't look well. I wondered if that was how I looked.

"Oh ya ... been there, done that. That's actually why I have this damn thing," David said, kicking his walker. "Too much Prednisone leaches calcium from your bones and turns them to shit."

My heart instantly hurt for David, and I felt ashamed for being so cold toward him. Up until that conversation, I had no idea that, in addition to making me a raging lunatic, Prednisone could affect my bones. Apparently, there was a lot I didn't know about the disease I'd been living with for over a decade. Mostly because I wasn't interested in finding out just how bad things could get. I figured the less I knew, the better. The less connection I felt to my disease, my body, and others with this disease, the better. It was a flawed plan rooted in fear.

I took a deep breath and decided to give this connection thing a try. "So, David ... what's your story?"

David was twenty-two; diagnosed with Crohn's disease when he was eleven. He had a three-year-old son, which surprised me because David seemed like a child himself. Earlier in the year, David had an ileostomy and recently started experiencing some complications. Hence, his most recent hospital stay.

"What's an ileostomy?" I was afraid to ask—and felt a little embarrassed for not knowing the answer.

"Girl! You have Crohn's and don't know what an ileostomy is?" David patted his belly as he explained that an ileostomy is a surgery that creates a hole in the abdomen wall and connects to a plastic bag on the outside of the body to collect waste. "It's the surgery you get for a shit bag. Do you want to see it?"

I thought I might actually pass out right then and there.

Did I want to see it? Abso-fucking-lutely not! I didn't want to see it, read about it, know about it, or think about it! Ugh—this opening up thing was a terrible idea! My heart started racing, and I began to feel hot and dizzy. How could David discuss his "shit bag" so casually, as if it were no big deal? As if he were proud of it or something! Jesus, I should never have left my room. This is exactly why I didn't want to attend the support groups or watch any ridiculous videos.

"I'll pass, but thanks for the offer."

David went on to tell me that his "baby mama" (his words, not mine) recently broke up with him. "Apparently, she had enough of caring for two people." It made me wonder if someday I would be too much of a burden for Joe and the girls.

In addition to being recently dumped, David was broke from all the medical bills. "I'm meeting with a social worker tomorrow to talk about applying for Medicaid." I felt myself begin to soften again as David painted a picture of his life. A life very different from my own—and yet, we both shared the same diagnosis.

"What about your folks?" I naïvely asked.

"Nah. We're not really close. It's cool though."

I couldn't imagine not having the support of my husband, family, and friends. I was lucky enough to have so many people who loved and rallied around me. They were all begging me to take care of myself, and I was selfishly poo-pooing them because I was too scared to face reality.

I took another breath and decided to keep walking with David. I told myself I could feel afraid but stay present and curious with my fear. We walked a few more laps around the floor before it was time to get hooked back up to my IV. It was the longest I had ever talked to another person with Crohn's disease about Crohn's disease in a serious way, in my entire life—including my very own sister. In those thirty minutes, I learned more about Crohn's and its many complications than I had in the past decade.

I returned to my room feeling overwhelmed, sad, and tired. There was no escaping the heavy darkness I felt. There were no emails to respond to or diapers to change. The only option I had was sleep. So, I went to the bathroom for the millionth time that day, hooked myself back up to my IV pole, turned off the light over my bed, and tried to forget about David and his bag.

* * *

I woke up hours later to a nurse standing over my bed. "Miss, it's time to wake up and prep for your CT scan." She handed me a large bottle of "oral prep," which is a thick, disgusting cocktail of barium and God-knows-what-else that tastes like death. "Drink the entire bottle and I'll come back in an hour to check on you."

After not eating for days, you would have thought my body would have welcomed something with a little more substance. I took three huge chugs and tried to convince myself I was drinking the world's most delicious vanilla milkshake.

But by the fourth gulp, I started to get really bloated and super nauseous. I instantly ran to the bathroom and relieved myself in the ridiculous poop hat. This was no milkshake. It was more like drinking thick liquid aspirin mixed with glue. I gagged, took another chug, and tried to breathe slowly so as not to throw up. The more I drank, the more bloated and uncomfortable I became. It took me a full ninety minutes to choke down the entire bottle.

Once I was done with the prep, I laid back down in my bed. I curled up in the fetal position, tummy gurgling, head pounding, and tried to drown out the sounds of my roommate, who was moaning in pain. All I wanted to do was go back to sleep.

"Please, someone help me," she groaned from behind the curtain, "I need help with my bag. Please."

"Ma'am ... do you need me to get the nurse?" Damnit! I did not want to get involved, but now I had no choice. The faceless woman behind the curtain sounded as if she were a wounded animal, and it terrified me.

More moans. "Yes please."

I rolled onto my side, untangled the tubes, grabbed my IV pole, and—with a sloshy stomach full of barium—headed to the nurses' station. The moment I stood up, I felt lightheaded and even more nauseous.

"I was wondering if you could help my roommate. She seems to be in a lot of pain." I willed myself to not throw up all over the nurses' station.

"Of course. Also, it's time for you to drink the second bottle of prep," the nurse said, handing me another huge bottle.

"I'm sorry, what? I have to drink *another* one of those?" It took everything in me to choke down the first bottle without throwing up. How in the world was I going to get another entire bottle of that crap inside me? It seemed impossible, and I started tearing up.

"Yes. You have to drink another bottle for the prep. If you don't drink enough, we won't be able to get a good contrast for the scan, and you'll have to do this all over again."

Maybe it was the hunger or that I missed my girls so much it hurt. Maybe it was the conversation with David earlier or the terrifying moans coming from behind the curtain in my room. Whatever it was, I instantly felt defeated and broken as I began to openly sob. I hated myself for acting like such a baby in front of her—for showing her what I perceived as weakness, which was really just my messy, vulnerable humanity.

"Oh honey, it's okay." The nurse got up from behind the desk and gently patted me on the back. "Just do your best. One sip at a time and it will be over before you know it." The feeling of connection ran through me again. It was warm and comforting and made me cry even harder.

We walked back to my room, and I thanked the nurse for her kindness. Then, I locked myself in the bathroom with the giant bottle of ick.

Alright, Chris ... it's go time. You can do this—just like bonging a beer in college.

Before I started choking down the rest of my prep, I looked at myself in the mirror for the first time since being admitted. I looked like a disheveled, greasy child. The dark circles under my eyes had turned even darker. My cheeks were sunken even more. The color of my skin was a putrid gray. My collarbones jutted out the top of my hospital gown. I hardly recognized myself. How had I let things get this bad?

I took a breath and said a prayer for the first time since I could remember. My grandmother, the one I spoke to a few days earlier, used to say that no prayer was too small—that God wanted us to lay our problems, of any size, before Him and humbly ask for help. At first, I felt foolish asking God to help me with something so insignificant as drinking a gallon of barium—when there were people, like David, with real problems. But I was desperate and willing to test my grandmother's "nothing is too small" theory. At that point, there was no way in hell I was getting the rest of that barium in me any other way. So, I turned that tiny bathroom into my own personal church and began to pray.

Then I opened the second bottle, took a sip, and instantly threw it back up into the sink.

Come on, God ... I'm here asking for help—the one thing I hate doing more than drinking this shit. Please. Help me. Please.

I took another sip. I gagged a little, but it stayed down. And then another. And another. And another. My stomach gurgled, and I relieved myself three more times in the poop hat. There was still blood. A lot of blood. My head was pounding, and my whole body hurt. I started crying again but continued drinking, with tears and snot running down my face.

One sip at a time.

One breath at a time.

One day at a time.

In that tiny cold bathroom, I began to realize there was no way out of this. There were no more places to hide. I could no longer ignore my physical, mental, and emotional health. I had to face reality and, as silly as it sounds, it started with me finishing that drink. I was going to have to take it—sip by bitter sip— until it was gone. There was no speeding through it. If I tried to chug it, I would throw up and have to start all over again.

I kept taking small, steady sips and continued to pray.

That disgusting drink taught me that sometimes we have to face the things in life that are bitter and hard to swallow; the things we would never willingly choose to carry with us but, for whatever reason, are ours to carry just the same. At that moment, I realized the biggest thing I was carrying wasn't my Crohn's; it was my fear. And I was crumbling under the weight of it.

I had become so afraid that I preferred to bury my head in the sand and tell everyone that I was fine—in the hope of convincing myself I actually was. I suddenly realized, "I'm fine" was the biggest lie I had ever told.

Instead of lying all these years, I should have just told the truth. I should have said, "Actually, I'm not fine. I'm scared, anxious, and depressed. I feel like my body just gave me the middle finger. I feel like it's all my fault. I feel like I let everyone down. And I'm exhausted and in pain most of the time, and as a result, I feel angry most of the time. I feel so angry I could scream at the top of my lungs, flip over a table, and attack the next person who looks at me sideways. No, I'm not fine. I am anything but."

Of course, I never said any of that. Instead, I swallowed down all of my pain, anger, and fear and let it make me even sicker. I was so afraid to take a long hard look at myself and admit there was something inside of me I would never be able to fix or cover up with a big smile, pretty dress, or fancy job.

I had to stop telling people I was fine when I clearly wasn't. I had to start empowering myself with knowledge and loving myself enough to receive the support that so many people were trying to extend. I had to realize—this is me. I am David. I am my roommate. I am living with a chronic disease and, by definition, will for the rest of my life.

So, now what?

"*I realized the biggest thing I was carrying wasn't my Crohn's; it was my fear.*"

CHAPTER 14

I'M NOT FINE

———

Shortly after my diagnosis in 1997, I started having a recurring dream about a hidden room.

The premise of the dream is always roughly the same: I'm walking around an empty building, school, or house. And while I've never been there before, there's something vaguely familiar about it—that I can't quite put my finger on.

I wander through the hallways alone and searching—for what, I'm not exactly sure. But there is an eerie knowing accompanying me on my journey. That eerie knowing is whispering to me, "There's more, keeping going, keep remembering, you're almost there."

Eventually, I stumble upon a hidden room. I can't ever recall what's in the room, but the feelings I experience when I walk inside are always the same.

I feel excited, happy, and full of radiant, warm light.

I'm enamored with the room each and every time. There's something special about it. It feels magical ... like when dawn breaks on Christmas morning or seeing the ocean for the first time. There's something waiting for me in that room. I can *feel* it. And all I want to do is sit in the middle of the room and drink in the warmth and peace I feel there.

And then, just as quickly as I stumble upon the room, it's gone. I'm back in the dark hallway alone, searching and a little afraid. I feel unsettled and spend the rest of the dream trying to get back to the hidden room that brought me so much comfort and joy. I search and search but can't seem to retrace my steps or find my way back before waking.

I had versions of that dream for years before I finally understood its significance.

The warmth and light and joy I felt in that room was me: the best, most authentic version of me—regardless of my diagnosis or what I looked like or achieved.

The unconscious grief I experienced after my diagnosis nearly nailed that room shut. Throughout the years, there would be times when the door cracked open just long enough for me to get a glimpse of the girl inside. That girl was confident, brave, and full of love and energy—palpable energy. She channeled her inner Angela Bower. She wasn't broken or sick, and she didn't play small. She didn't need to. She could be as big and bold as she wanted and didn't have to apologize for—or fear—her body or the world around her.

The little girl inside that room is who I was searching for in my dream all those years. She was in there, waiting for me to return.

* * *

I left the hospital a week later, no better than when I arrived. Six days of intravenous steroids and a liquid diet to calm my digestive system hadn't worked. I lost fourteen pounds and was so weak I couldn't walk up the steps to my bedroom once I got home, so I slept on the living room couch for a few nights.

My body was clearly waving the white flag. She started speaking to me:

Enough is enough, Chris. We can't go on like this anymore. You're exhausted. I'm exhausted. We've tried your way for years, and it's just not working. So now we are going to try another way ... the Universe's way. You remember the Universe, don't you? That light inside of you? I know you do. That's what you've been dreaming about in that hidden room all these years. I've been visiting you in that dream over and over again, trying to get you to remember who you really are. You are not undeserving, bad, shameful, gross, broken, or a monster. You're that little girl who used to play and dream in that room. You are full of love, goodness, and energy. Let's go find her and let her shine again.

That week in the hospital was a wake-up call and turning point. After working through the peak of my resistance, denial, and rage, I realized I had made an enemy out of my body for far too long. I had turned my back on her for being different. She wasn't broken. I wasn't broken. We were both sad and not fully aware of the other. I needed to learn how to stop fleeing and fighting my body ... I needed to befriend it.

Something had to change. Actually, a lot had to change, and it was no one's responsibility but mine. It was time I faced my fears and heeded the advice I heard for years. I needed to "go into the woods" like I did as a child with my mom and, quite frankly, ... slow the hell down.

When I returned home from the hospital, I felt a shift occur deep within me. I recently spoke with my husband about this period of our marriage, my illness, and the toll all that running took on us both. He used the word "shredded" to describe my condition after I left the hospital. "You were so weak. It was almost as if you were elderly."

Joe was right. I was shredded, both physically and emotionally—and, for the first time since I was diagnosed, I allowed myself to properly grieve. I laid on my couch and cried and journaled, and then cried some more.

Reality was finally sinking in. Yes, I was sick. No, I couldn't fix it. But I wasn't powerless either. I had choices. I always had choices—and it was time I started choosing myself.

During a follow-up appointment a few days after I got out of the hospital, my doctor told me that I had to make a choice between toxic medication (that could cause cancer or medically induced Lupus) or undergo surgery to have my entire colon and rectum removed, and likely live with a bag the rest of my life. I sobbed the entire drive home from my doctor's.

Turns out I was sick. Really sick. And everyone knew it but me. Or maybe I did know it and didn't want to believe it. I thought if I kept hiding and running and moving and smiling and lying that my disease wouldn't find me. But she always did, like a child seeking attention. *Look at me! Notice me! Why won't you talk to me?*

The longer I ignored her, the louder she became—until I could no longer pretend I didn't hear her. The truth is I had been sad and angry for over a decade and was carrying so much pain that I didn't even realize just how bad things had become. But there I was left with only two choices: more medication or surgery—neither of which I wanted to make.

But what if there was another option? What if I started telling the truth? My truth. Yes, I'm in pain. Yes, I'm exhausted. Yes, I am losing so much blood every time I go to the bathroom that I'm afraid to look because it feels like evidence of my body failing me. Yes, I need help. Yes, I need rest. Yes, I surrender.

Little by little, all of those small truths started to tear down the wall of lies I had built around me. And little by little, I began to heal physically and emotionally.

During this time, a friend gave me a copy of the book *A Return to Love* by Marianne Williamson, and it changed my life. I've read this book countless times and have highlighted, underlined, and dog-eared practically the entire thing. I used to carry it in my purse until the spine broke and the cover fell off. Now I keep it on my nightstand and return to it whenever I feel my fear rising.

In *A Return to Love*, Williamson writes:

To trust in the force that moves the universe is faith. Faith isn't blind, it's visionary. Faith is believing that the universe is on our side, and that the universe knows what it's doing. Faith is a psychological awareness of an unfolding force for good, constantly at work in all dimensions. Our attempts to direct this force only interferes with it. Our willingness to relax in to it allows it to work on our behalf. Without faith, we're frantically trying to control what is not ours to control, and fix what is not in our power to fix. What we're trying to control is much better off without us, and what we're trying to fix can't be fixed by us anyway. Without faith, we're wasting time.

I had, in fact, wasted time by fighting against, downplaying, and turning my disease into an enemy. My Crohn's was not something for me to control and fight against; it was something inside me that needed love and attention. In order to make that shift from fear to love, I needed to start by being honest with myself.

I was not fine.

I was terrified.

I was devastated.

I was heartbroken.

I was angry.

It was time to stop running and hiding—and finally start telling the truth.

"It was time to stop running and hiding—and finally start telling the truth."

CHAPTER 15

THE FOURTH F

——

Not once since I was diagnosed with Crohn's did I ever consider actually loving my body as is. But that's exactly what was needed ... radical, unconditional self-love. (Thank you, Sonya Renee Taylor!)

I was introduced to Sonya Renee Taylor while listening to *Brené* Brown's podcast *Unlocking Us*. The two women connected because of a quote that went viral during the COVID-19 shutdown; that was mistakenly attributed to *Brené* but was actually Sonya's:

"We will not go back to normal. Normal never was. Our pre-corona existence was never normal other than we normalized greed, inequity, exhaustion, depletion, extraction, disconnection, confusion, rage, hoarding, hate, and lack. We should not long to return, my friends. We are being given the opportunity to stitch a new garment. One that fits all of humanity and nature."

Even more beautiful than Sonya's quote was the discussion they had about her book *The Body Is Not an Apology: The Power of Radical Self-Love*.

Listening to the conversation, I was stunned and deeply affected. If you haven't listened to the podcast, I implore you—immediately download and listen to the September 16, 2020, episode of *Unlocking Us*. (You can thank me later!)

As someone with a chronic disease and deep-rooted body image issues, Sonya's message had me nodding my head "Yes" the entire time. I never heard anyone so perfectly capture what it felt like to live in a body that was different. I took her message one step further. Not only is my body *not an apology*, it's also not an enemy or a failure.

For years after my diagnosis, I turned my body into an enemy that I fought against every day. I was mad at my body for what I perceived as it failing and attacking me. I was mad at my body for not working or looking the way I wanted it to.

I didn't love or trust my body for nearly half my life, so how did I expect it to love or trust me back? I took my body for granted in so many ways and trained myself to disconnect from it whenever possible.

For years I had the hardest time crying or expressing emotions other than toxic positivity on one end of the spectrum or rage on the other end. To express emotions accurately, I needed to be in my body and feel my feelings. I refused to be in my body for years, and the consequences of that behavior finally caught up with me. There was nowhere left to run. There was no one left to fight.

I was faced with a choice: continue to carry this anger and self-hatred until it sunk my health, my marriage, and myself completely, or decide to feel it all and acknowledge that my body is not—and never was—an apology, enemy, or failure.

And while I didn't know exactly how I would go about making these changes, I knew the first step was to stop numbing and start feeling—to start remembering who I was before I let fear become my primary motivator.

I needed to reframe and see my disease for what it was and was not. What if Crohn's wasn't a villain trying to destroy me, but rather, a small child seeking love and attention? What if I could make friends with my body: love her and care for her like I do my own children?

There is a section at the end of *A Return to Love* where Marianne Williamson writes about health and healing that blew my mind and broke my heart wide open. In it, she writes: *"Love changes the way we think about our disease. Of course, people hate their cancer ... but the last thing a sick person needs is something else to hate about themselves. Healing results from a transformed perception of our relationship to illness, one in which we respond to the problem with love instead of fear."*

Love my Crohn's disease? After all that jerk has put me through. Even if I need surgery and an ostomy bag? That's a tall order, Marianne. How is that even possible? She continues:

"If I'm yelling, the person in front of me can react in one of two ways. He can yell back, screaming at me to shut up, but this will tend to make me scream more. Or he can tell me that he cares what my feelings are, and he loves me and is sorry that I'm feeling this way, which will tend to quiet me down. Those are our two choices with critical illness."

She goes on to say that attacking our disease will not lead to a cure, and that approach will only make it grow stronger and louder. "Healing comes from entering into a conversation with our illness, seeking to understand what it's trying to tell us."

Well, well, well. Looks like I had been going about this the wrong way. No wonder my body was so pissed at me and decided enough was enough. I was either screaming my head off at her or giving her the total silent treatment—for over a decade. She was tired of being ignored and pushed aside. And, like a child yearning for love and attention, she decided that the only way to get my attention was to act out.

So much about my body felt out of my control, and for the most part, a lot of it was. Although I would never be able to control the circumstances of my diagnosis, I could control my perception and reaction to it. I could start telling the truth. I could stop punishing myself. I could start feeling and finally grieve out in the open. I could start admitting that although I was powerless over my diagnosis, I was absolutely not powerless in how I lived life with my diagnosis. It would be a process, and it wouldn't happen overnight. But how?

The phrase "One day at a time" kept ringing in my ears as I thought about my cousin, Sarah.

* * *

Growing up, I idolized my older cousin, Sarah. After she went through a brief tomboy phase, she transformed into what I perceived as the coolest, most beautiful teenager in the whole world. She traded in her soccer shorts for Janet Jackson-esque outfits and had big hair held in place by Aussie hairspray. She even had a signature color ... purple (hence the Aussie hairspray that smells like grape and comes in a huge purple can). When she insisted on only using purple pens, I insisted too. She was like the big sister I never had, and I hung on her every word.

Something started to happen to Sarah in high school: another transformation. She went from tomboy to girly-girl to addict in front of my eyes. And while her story is not mine to tell, what I can share, with her permission, is her healing. By the time Sarah was sixteen, she had completed a stint in rehab, got sober, and has been for over twenty years.

Her sobriety didn't happen by accident. It happened because she accepted her disease, surrendered to a higher power, and took responsibility for it every single day, one day at a time. She started attending Alcoholics Anonymous, got a sponsor, set boundaries, and avoided triggering situations and toxic people. She realized she could not achieve lasting sobriety on her own. She needed others. She needed faith. She needed herself.

The week after I got out of the hospital, I thought a lot about Sarah—and something clicked. What if I treated my disease and quest for remission the way she treated her addiction and quest for sobriety? What if I set time aside every day to work toward remission? It would require me to be vigilant, ask for help, surrender, and—above all else—start loving myself by taking care of my mind, body, and spirit.

Would it be easy? Hell no. Would it be worth it? Absofrickin-lutely, because my life depended on it. I was ready and willing to try a different way. But first, I needed to do the one thing I never properly did all those years ago—I needed to grieve.

A few weeks ago, I had a fascinating conversation with an acquaintance from high school named Janelle. We had reconnected through Facebook, and I was so excited to speak with her again after all these years. I remembered Janelle as such a kind, genuine, warm person and wasn't surprised in the least that she grew up to become a counselor.

We talked about the difference between traditional PTSD (Posttraumatic Stress Disorder) and illness-induced PTSD: something I had never heard of prior to our conversation but realized is exactly what I was experiencing from age seventeen to twenty-nine.

Because chronic illness is well ... *chronic* ... by definition, there is no fixed endpoint. And because illness is an internal versus an external threat, such as war or abuse, there is no escaping it, which can make illness-induced PTSD a little tricky. Symptoms can include anxiety, difficulties sleeping, shame and self-blame, withdrawal from social situations, and treatment avoidance. Sound familiar?

According to a study published in *Frontline Gastroenterology*, 19 percent of patients with Crohn's disease screened positive for a PTSD diagnosis. As a point of comparison, 11–20 percent of military veterans have PTSD.

And guess what is required in order to heal from illness-induced PTSD? You guessed it ... grieving.

"Grief is a different kind of pain. There's good pain, there's bad pain, and then there's grief. Grief is the letting go and processing of something. It requires a radical acceptance of what's going on in order to enter into the grieving process and begin to heal," Janelle explained.

The week after I left the hospital, I took the first step on my journey to radical acceptance. I made a lot of progress that next year, but radical acceptance is something that requires ongoing practice.

Here's what it looked like for me:

RADICAL ACCEPTANCE #1:

Crohn's disease is a chronic illness for which there is no cure, and I must accept that it will always be a part of my life. I must also accept that I will be on medication for the rest of my life, regardless of if I'm flaring or not. I must accept that my body operates differently than others, and I will have to worry about things I'd rather not think about—like side effects, procedures, and medical bills—for the rest of my life. As one doctor told me, "Crohn's is like a diamond; it's forever." Radical Acceptance #1 was the toughest pill I had to swallow in over a decade. But it was time ... down the hatch!

RADICAL ACCEPTANCE #2:

Crohn's disease affects my mental and emotional health, and anti-anxiety medication is super beneficial. Sometimes my diagnosis makes me feel sad and overwhelmed, and other times, anxious and scared. These feelings do not make me a weak, bad, or ungrateful person; they make me human. For me, mental and emotional health greatly impact my symptoms—and it is my responsibility to keep both in check.

RADICAL ACCEPTANCE #3:

I need to start telling the truth to myself and others. I am not invincible, and I can't do it all. Regardless of how I look on the outside, I'm not fine all the time. There will be days and weeks I need a little extra help and support. There will be days I feel like garbage. No more downplaying, minimizing, or self-gaslighting. No more saying "yes" when I really want to say "no" just to make others feel comfortable. My own comfort and care must come first, and if people are disappointed, so be it.

RADICAL ACCEPTANCE #4:

I have to slow down and sit with hard feelings instead of sprinting away from them. I must accept the fact that my body requires more rest than someone without an autoimmune disease. This doesn't mean I'm lazy, unmotivated, or overly dramatic.

RADICAL ACCEPTANCE #5:

It is my responsibility to care for and advocate for my body, mind, and spirit. It is no one's job but mine to take my medicine as prescribed, stay on top of my doctor's appointments, be more mindful of what I'm putting in my body, and rid myself of toxic people and situations that do not serve my best interests. I am empowered in whatever moment I empower *myself*. I must stop waiting for permission to take better care of myself and start making it a priority.

That first week out of the hospital, my eyes were opened for the first time in over a decade. I couldn't believe how bad I let things get. And I made myself promise to never let them get that bad again.

It was time to start making some changes.

"I didn't love or trust my body for nearly half my life, so how did I expect it to love or trust me back?"

PART 3 JOURNAL PROMPTS:

———

- Have you ever downplayed or hid your symptoms from your friends, family, or physicians? If so, why? What would happen if you told the truth?
- Have you ever had a "brick wall moment" related to your illness or condition? What happened? How will you prevent "brick wall moments" in the future?
- Write a letter to your chronic illness or condition and your current relationship. What are you afraid of most? What do you appreciate most? Do you need to make amends? If so, how will you?

PART 4

(BE)FRIENDING

CHAPTER 16

CHANGES (PART 1)

———

After my hospital stay, I had a lot of processing and soul-searching to do.

Clearly, I had a lot of fear. I was afraid to acknowledge how serious this disease could be and the potential impact it could have on my life. I was afraid of being different, and I was afraid of slowing down for fear of never getting back up.

So, there you have it. I was a big, fat scaredy-cat and had to make a decision. Did I want to continue being afraid and fighting against myself for the rest of my life, or did I want to face my reality with grace, love, and care? An auto-immune disease is literally the body fighting against itself. What if I called a truce? No more fighting against myself. I had enough of that happening already, and quite frankly, I deserved better.

I kept coming back to a line I read in *A Return to Love* about the true definition of the word miracle, which is a shift in perspective "from fear to love." I needed to quit fearing myself and all the things about my body I couldn't control and replace that energy with love.

I had been living in fear since I was a teenager. The eating disorder, the self-gaslighting, the insatiable need to please and prove myself, the inability to set boundaries, not properly caring for myself ... all of myself ... were evidence of a fearful lifestyle. Let's face it, whether I had a chronic medical condition or not, this fear-based living was my OG chronic condition from way back in the day when I was afraid of ticks and tornados.

My fear was like gasoline on a fire, and it was time to start living in love instead of fear. It's not easy to love something about ourselves we wish was different ... no one *wants* to deal with chronic illness. But if this was my reality, it was time to lay my weapons down and let love lead the way—which leads me to Change #1:

CHANGE #1: WAKE UP & SURRENDER

First and foremost, I needed to wake up and stop avoiding things that made me uncomfortable or scared in the hope they would magically disappear on their own. The Universe tested me early on to see just how serious I was about this change.

One morning—about a week or so after I got out of the hospital—I was lying in bed when my husband rolled over and pulled down my tank top a little. I smiled, knowing what that meant. But when I opened my eyes, he had a concerned look on his face. "Chris, what is that?" he asked, pointing to the spot between my sternum and right breast. I had lost even more weight during my week in the hospital, and you could literally see every bone in my chest.

"What is what?" I said, blinking sleep out of my eyes.

"That lump, I can see it. Have you not noticed it?"

I reached down and felt the area Joe was pointing to—and my heart stopped. Somehow, between the follow-up appointments and additional tests for my Crohn's, I honestly hadn't noticed the huge lump that had formed on my right breast.

My first thought was, "No fucking way. I have enough to deal with right now. I don't need this, too." The urge to hide instantly bubbled up.

"Chris, you have to call the doctor TODAY," he insisted, instantly sensing my fear. Damn it, he knew me too well!

Guess who avoided calling the doctor for three full days?

It all felt like too much to deal with, on top of what I was currently going through with my Crohn's. My brain didn't have the capacity to process the lump on top of the bomb my doctor dropped about potentially living the rest of my life without a colon or rectum. For a moment, I started to shut down. But then I remembered Sarah and her daily commitment to her sobriety.

One day at a time, Chris. Come on, you can do this. No more hiding, remember?

It was literally the last thing I wanted to deal with, but I knew this was my chance to start walking the talk. No more burying my head in the sand and pretending scary things like a toilet full of blood and large, visible lumps on my breast didn't exist. Neither one of those things would ever resolve themselves by me ignoring them.

It was time to stand my ground and stare down my fear. In that moment, I realized it is perfectly okay and entirely possible to be terrified and do something anyways.

I went to see my general doctor the next day. After examining my breast, he ordered what felt like my four hundredth X-ray that year. The results of the X-ray resulted in a biopsy of the lump—and the biopsy of the lump resulted in surgery. Each call from my doctor's office made my heart stop as I wondered, is this the call where I learn I have Crohn's disease *and* breast cancer?

"Since the results of your biopsy came back inconclusive, the doctor would like to schedule you for a lumpectomy as soon as possible." The nurse explained to me this was the only way to definitely rule out cancer.

"Okay. What does that mean?" I asked, afraid to find out.

I took a deep breath and let out a long exhale like I did when I smoked those trashy Marlboro Lights. A month prior, I was in the hospital praying I wouldn't need surgery on my colon—only to find out I needed a different kind of surgery altogether. I should have been terrified and supremely anxious, but this time I wasn't. And it's not because I was in denial. I simply refused to worry until I had something to worry about. At that moment, all I had was a benign lump.

That's when I said the most important prayer I have ever and will ever say. Four little words that came to me in that moment of despair and uncertainty: *I surrender, lead me.*

So simple, yet so powerful.

"I surrender" doesn't mean we ignore and hide our pain. It means we show up for ourselves with love and compassion and then surrender the situation to a higher power, the universe, God ... whatever term floats your spiritual boat.

"Lead me" doesn't mean we throw our hands up in the air and wait for some mystical sign to show us the way. It means we trust that we will be led to what we need most at any given moment. "I surrender, lead me" replaced "I'm fine" as my new rallying cry. And the amazing thing was, unlike "I'm fine," I *actually* meant it.

I said it as I called to schedule my lumpectomy. *I surrender, lead me.*

I said it when I kissed Joe goodbye and got wheeled back to the operating room. *I surrender, lead me.*

I said it days later when my phone lit up with my doctor's name, calling to share the results of my surgery. *I surrender, lead me.* Whatever my doctor was about to tell me, I would surrender and trust that I would be led through it somehow, some way. I didn't need to have all the answers. I only needed to let go and have faith that no matter the outcome, I would be okay. There is great peace that comes with surrender. Make no mistake, surrender is not passive. It's incredibly powerful and helps us to remember the "Serenity Prayer" that is so popular in Alcoholics Anonymous:

Grant me the serenity to accept the things I cannot change, the courage to change the things I can, and the wisdom to know the difference.

You know ... one day at a time.

Thankfully, I did not have cancer. I let out a huge sigh of relief and immediately shared the good news with Joe. As he was holding me, I had a realization: I was a hell of a lot stronger than I ever gave myself credit for, and it was about time I started realizing it. It felt oddly empowering to face something so terrifying head-on. Turns out, all I needed to do was surrender.

"I surrender, lead me."

CHAPTER 17

CHANGES (PART 2)

Once I realized the power of Change #1, I started feeling a little braver and was ready to make more changes. There was one change I knew I had needed to make for years, but that scared the shit out of me ... sometimes quite literally. That change was emotional awareness and honesty.

Ugh. I had been avoiding this one like the plague for years. Emotional honesty never really felt safe for me. It felt like something overly dramatic people did, and I wasn't interested in feeling or articulating anything other than pleasantries. What was the harm in swallowing negative emotions? Isn't that what nice girls do? Isn't that what my parents raised me to do?

The harm, of course, was every time I avoided or denied an uncomfortable emotion or conversation, it made me sick. Every time I said I was fine when I wasn't, it made me sick. Every time I politely said "Yes," when all I really wanted to say was "Hell no," it made me sick.

I could not control my diagnosis, but I absolutely could control the amount of emotional poison I was ingesting every day. If I was going to take my quest for remission seriously, I needed to start telling the truth as if my life depended on it ... because it kind of did. At the very least, my colon and rectum did.

This is something I started practicing little by little in those early years after I got out of the hospital. I started small by promising myself to simply tell the truth when someone asked me how I was doing. No more "grin and bear it" mentality. Time to get down to brass tacks. So, when a mom from Stella's school called me a month after I got out of the hospital and asked how I was doing, I decided to try out this whole emotional honesty thing.

I took a deep breath and decided to just tell the truth. "How am I doing? Honestly, not great. I'm actually physically exhausted and emotionally overwhelmed." There. I said it. She could run away in disgust and discomfort if she wanted to, but at least I told the truth.

And then something incredible happened. She didn't recoil in horror as I thought ... quite the opposite. My emotional honesty opened a door for her emotional honesty to waltz through. Apparently, she was feeling the same way but for different reasons. We spent the next hour having an honest conversation, and both wondered why we had never talked about these kinds of things before.

"I know why," I said, holding the phone while making peanut butter and jelly sandwiches for the girls. "It's because we were afraid of not appearing put together. We were afraid of making each other uncomfortable and being judged for not being perfect. Do you feel uncomfortable or judged?"

"No, I actually feel like a huge weight has been lifted," she replied. "I've been bottling up all this stress for weeks and felt like I was going to explode if I didn't get it out. Thanks for listening. I feel one hundred times better."

I really liked the idea of feeling one hundred times better, and if that small exchange was what emotional honesty could lead to, I was here for it.

Let's be clear, this is still really hard for me and something I struggle with to this day. Old habits die hard, and it's easy for me to slip back into being an emotional fibber—as I did in 2016, after my family experienced a house fire.

Thank goodness no one was hurt, but the experience itself was terrifying and traumatic. Knowing how close my family was to danger, knowing how fleeting life could be, knowing how randomly tragedy could strike really shook me. As a result of that experience, I relapsed into hiding from those really big, really scary emotions. That is—until I learned a little trick a few years ago during a therapy session.

CHANGE #2: NOTICE THE LUMPS

I notice my lump. (No, not the one in my breast, although that is just as important.) The one in my throat.

The one I prefer to shove down and swallow the moment I'm faced with an emotionally uncomfortable or vulnerable situation. "I'm fine" created that lump in my throat, and the only way to break it up was to start telling the truth. I was unsure how to be emotionally honest until I started listening to my body and noticing how it felt when I lied.

If you're a people-pleaser by nature, try noticing what happens in your body when you are being emotionally dishonest. Maybe your shoulders tense up, or your jaw tightens. However, it shows up in your body, I can promise you this much—that pain is a physical manifestation of your lie. It's what emotional dishonesty ultimately leads to ... pain and suffering. And don't we have enough of that to deal with already?

I didn't recognize my telltale sign until I sat in front of my therapist, Koren, a few years ago, right after the fire. She taught me how to listen to my body, which, as you know, was something I avoided for years.

I sat down on the couch in Koren's office as we began the intake process. "What brings you in today?" Her voice was gentle and soothing, exactly what you would expect from a therapist who specializes in trauma.

My first reaction was to downplay and make light of the situation. "Oh God ... where do I start?"

Koren just looked at me patiently in silence. We were playing emotional chicken, and there was no way this lady was going to let me swerve. I took a breath and tried to just say something honest and true, "I guess it's just that I feel scared a lot of the time."

I told her about the house fire and could feel my heart start to beat faster. Just saying the word "*fire*" made my body buzz and my throat hurt. "I also think I'm turning into a workaholic. I feel like I can't stop thinking about work. I'm afraid if I do, I'll make a mistake." I took a sip of water and started to fan myself with my hand. Jesus, it was hot in her office.

"Or worse ... my boss and coworkers will find out what a fraud I am, and I'll get fired. And then everything will fall apart, and my family will be homeless. I know that sounds extreme, but the fear of failure has such a chokehold on me, and it's all related to my career."

Koren smiled. "Is it really all just related to your career?"

I told her I didn't know but that I just couldn't seem to ever shut work off. "I feel like I'm sprinting all day every day and can't stop. I wake up at 2 a.m. and start obsessively researching various work-related topics. Then I wake up and do it all over again. I swear if I didn't have a family to come home to, I would have no problem working until nine o'clock every night."

"On the weekends, I feel restless, agitated but exhausted. Like I don't know exactly what to do with myself." I was on a roll now. "And I'm tired. So fucking tired. But I can't let myself sit or rest. I imagine it's like being on cocaine, although I've never actually done it. I feel like I'm constantly buzzing and can't turn my brain or body off." I was full-on sweating now. I just had verbal diarrhea all over her couch—and somehow felt more uncomfortable admitting all of that to a total stranger than if I had *actually* had diarrhea on her couch.

She smiled and told me she understood exactly what I meant, "So, do you want to do the work?"

I shook my head "Yes," but had no clue what "the work" entailed. I was about to find out.

"Something tells me this goes back further than the fire. I'm sensing layers of trauma."

Busted.

"Ya. I think you're right."

"Alright then—let's get to work!" She was excited, and I was terrified. This "work" sounded messy.

And it was messy in the best way possible. The "work" changed my life and broke open my spirit in such a necessary way. It was hard because "the work" involved being in my body, fully present, and get this ... *feeling.* And then naming those my messy feelings. And then feeling those messy feelings I was naming. And I had to do it ... in front of her! As someone who was expertly trained in the fine art of "grin and bear it," this felt like a personal attack.

First, she tried something called EMDR (Eye Movement Desensitization and Reprocessing), which is a form of therapy used to treat people with PTSD. No such luck; because at the time, I was so incapable of being vulnerable with my eyes open. Having someone witness all my messy feelings up close and personal felt impossible to bear. No effing way.

"I don't think this is working," I said, fidgeting with my dress and avoiding eye contact with her. "It's like I can't fully access my feelings when you're looking at me. I can't let my guard down." Telling another mom at school that I was feeling overwhelmed and tired after getting out of the hospital was one thing. This shit was next level.

"Okay, let's try something else." She turned the lights down in her office and put on some quiet music. She told me to close my eyes and to take a deep breath. And then another. And then another. She gave me ice packs because I was so hot, which I learned is a trauma response. "Breathe. Get inside your body. What do you notice?"

"Um ... what do you mean? Like, what do I notice in the room?" I was trained to focus on the outside world.

"Not outside—inside. What do you notice happening inside your body at this moment? What's rising up? What are you feeling? And where?"

I squinted with my eyes closed, and I told her I wasn't sure.

"It's okay. Take another breath. Take your time. You're safe." In that moment, I actually believed her.

Just let go, Chris. Try. That's why you came here. Feel. Feel. What are you feeling? She said you were safe. Safe to feel in this dark room.

That's when I noticed the lump. "My throat feels tight."

"Good. What else?" She was treading lightly.

"It hurts and feels like there is an Indiana-Jones-sized boulder in there, and it's hard to swallow. It's actually getting worse." *Jesus, it's so hot in here.*

Koren leaned forward in her chair. "Good. You're doing really good. Can you go to that lump in your throat?"

I focused all my energy on the lump. It began pulsing and felt sharp, like shards of glass.

"Are you there?"

I nodded my head.

"And what are you feeling?"

I told her I felt pain, and she asked me if I could name what emotion was attached to the pain. I began to smile—my go-to response when any negative emotion starts rising. For a moment, the pain attempted to retreat, and I told myself it's not worth feeling, that this exercise was stupid and wasn't going to help.

Then the pain returned. It felt like an entire bag of Pop Rocks candy was stuck in my throat.

It took me a full minute before I realized what that pain feels like. It was suddenly so obvious. "It feels like I need to cry."

"And what *emotion* comes to mind when you think of crying?" She gently reminded me that crying isn't an emotion. It's something we do in response to an emotion.

"Um ..." My mind went blank, and I started getting frustrated with myself. *Come on, Chris, this isn't a test. It should be easy. What are you feeling? Just name an emotion. Why can't I name a goddamn emotion?*

"I know this isn't easy. Take a breath. What are you feeling?"

"Sad, I guess." My voice was barely louder than a whisper because the lump had grown so big and dense. It felt like someone had their hands around my neck and was trying to choke me to death.

"Good. Take another breath. When you think of feeling sad, what's the first thing that comes to mind?" This time she leaned back in her chair as if to give me space to examine and feel my heavy sadness.

"I know it sounds silly ... but being diagnosed with Crohn's disease makes me feel sad."

"It's not silly at all. That must have been hard." Her validation felt good. "Can you go back to the moment you were diagnosed? How old were you? What do you see? What do you remember?"

The lump was pushing against my throat harder than ever. It was trying its damnedest to silence me.

I told her that I see my seventeen-year-old self sitting on a table in my doctor's office, waiting for my test results. I feel my parents nervously watching me. I can sense their fear, and it scares me. In that moment, I'm more afraid of their reaction to my diagnosis than the diagnosis itself.

My therapist told me to go to my seventeen-year-old self as my thirty-seven-year-old self, sit next to her, and hold her hand.

"Okay. I'm sitting next to her. She's nervous and scared. She doesn't want to cause her parents pain or worry. She doesn't want them to be disappointed in her." I inhaled another deep breath. *Fuck, this is hard.* "After the doctor came in and confirmed my diagnosis, I felt myself disconnect. I told myself it was fine and not to be upset."

"But you were upset, weren't you?" I nodded my head and bit hard on my quivering bottom lip. "What would you tell that seventeen-year-old girl now? Go to her. What did she need to hear then, that none of the adults told her?"

Breathe, Chris. This is your chance. What would you tell her? Don't let that lump in your throat silence you anymore. It's been twenty years. Haven't you swallowed all of this down long enough? It's not working anymore. Think. What would you tell her?

And then it came to me: "I would tell her ... it's not your fault."

And with those four words, the lump began to crack wide open, and tears poured out of my eyes so effortlessly—even though I was sitting in front of a total stranger. Streams of tears watered the dry, painful lump in my throat, slowly melting it like hot water over an ice cube.

Holy shit, it's not my fault? It's not my fault! It never was! She handed me a box of tissues. "Why did you think it was your fault?"

"I thought God was punishing me for not being good enough. That I was bad or must have done something wrong." I was full-on ugly crying at that point. Snot, tears, snorting ... the whole bit.

I opened my eyes to see my therapist looking at me with pride and compassion. "Is that true?"

"God no. But I thought it was for the past twenty years. And I was carrying it with me morning, noon, and night— without ever realizing it." I couldn't help but laugh. "Holy shit, you're good!" My therapist laughed at my candor, and with that, our time together ended. And my adult life felt like it had finally begun.

Once I realized what that lump in my throat represented, I could no longer ignore it. That lump is my signal that something is wrong, and I'm not being honest with myself or others. There are some people that depended on that lump staying lodged firmly in place. Those people are slowly getting weeded out of my life.

I know that for me, the choice is binary: Ignore the lump, and let it choke me to death; or break it up, feel it, and realize things like, "It's not your fault."

Noticing the lump the moment it rises, is key. It's my clue to start feeling and paying attention, to be curious and scan my body for emotion instead of hibernating and hiding from it. Hibernation keeps me sick. Feeling is healing. That lump is my warning sign. Or, as Oprah would say, it's my whisper before the brick wall.

And I'm no longer interested in brick walls.

"It's not your fault."

CHAPTER 18

CHANGES (PART 3)

———

Pre-hospital stay, I was overextended and over-functioning (two of my very favorite hiding places) and had no one to blame but myself. I realized I had said yes to a lot of things in my life, not because I wanted to, but because it was a hell of a lot easier than saying no.

First of all, at that time, telling someone no felt really uncomfortable and selfish. I wanted people to like me, and in my mind, the straightest line to acceptance and love was agreeability. The problem with that myopic, fear-based view is that I was swapping my own feelings, needs, and comfort for someone else's—which is just one big, dangerous emotional fib.

Secondly, I didn't know how to say no without feeling an immense amount of guilt, so I often swapped it with a resentful yes. This clearly was not serving me because all of these inauthentic yesses left me exhausted and anxious with very little time to take care of my health.

CHANGE #3: BOUNDARIES

Once I started noticing the lump, I knew there was one more change I needed to make ... setting boundaries.

The first step in this new boundary-setting journey was making the difficult decision to change jobs. I was working in an environment and for a person who seriously lacked boundaries in and outside of work.

My boss at the time was a beautiful, smart, and charismatic woman whose approval I desperately wanted. As a result, I overlooked and made excuses for her inappropriate behavior for almost two years. This included, but was not limited to: her emotionally leaning on me while she had an affair with a married man, asking me to sign a non-compete clause (which is a legal document) after a night of drinking with clients, and cracking a beer *while driving* to a work function, after I told her it made me feel uncomfortable.

But after I found myself in the hospital for the fourth time in six months, I knew that environment, that job, and her leadership style were not serving me. Quite the opposite—it was literally making me sick. For the sake of my health, my sanity, and my rectum—I had to leave.

When you first start to set boundaries, it isn't easy, especially when the person with whom you are setting the boundary starts trying to negotiate with you—which is exactly what my former boss tried to do when she offered to give me a thirty-thousand-dollar raise if I stayed. Which was a lot more than the job I was leaving for.

For a moment, I wavered and started to second-guess myself. Then I took a breath and noticed how my body felt at the thought of staying in that job. And it didn't feel good. My body started buzzing, and I began to feel queasy. My colon was worth a hell of a lot more than thirty thousand dollars.

I stood up, shook her hand, politely thanked her, and said, "I wouldn't stay if you tripled my salary," and walked out of her office. It was kind of a mic-drop moment, and I have never felt so empowered in my entire career.

Was I afraid? Of course! But like most lessons I was learning, being afraid is never a good enough reason to stay in an unhealthy or limiting environment. And luckily, my first act of boundary-setting paid off big time.

I found myself working in a new environment—with people and products I truly loved. I felt supported and guided with healthy professional boundaries securely in place. When I left my job, I took a step back financially, and it was the best decision I ever made. Within a period of nine years, I had, in fact, tripled my income and was healthier than I'd ever been. In fact, I didn't have another flare-up for nearly five years ... which was the longest I'd ever been in remission.

This first foray into boundary-setting and emotional honesty gave me the confidence to just keep going no matter how big or small the situation. It just takes practice and consistency. Sure, I slip up from time to time, and the closer I am to someone, the harder it is for me—but I'm committed to making an effort every single day.

Here is a small example. I used to get asked all the time to join nonprofit committees or lead events at the girls' school. I hated saying no because I didn't want to disappoint anyone, and I felt like I *should* say yes. So, I would, and then I would feel anxious and resentful for taking on more than I could or wanted to handle.

"*Should*" is a tricky word. The moment it pops into my mind or out of someone else's mouth, I pause and recognize what's really going on ... manipulation by way of guilt. "*Should* I do something" or "Do I *want to* do something?" are two completely different things.

One day, a mom in Stella's class innocently asked if I would be willing to organize and lead the school bake sale. Before, I would have said an overly enthusiastic yes and then regretted it until the damn bake sale was over. This was my chance to practice my boundary-setting. I asked myself, "Do I feel like I *should* lead the bake sale, or do I *want* to lead the bake sale?"

As much as it pains me to admit, the answer was no. No, I never want to lead a bake sale. Or organize the class Valentine's Day party. Or head the school fundraiser.

No thank you—not after working all week long, keeping up on family activities, and trying to manage a chronic illness. What I *want* to do is be an individual contributor to the bake sale, the class party, and any other fundraiser—and am happy to do so.

And no, Karen, I will not be making organic homemade cookies and individually wrapping them in cute cellophane bags with raffia ribbons!

What I will be doing is hitting up the grocery store the morning of the bake sale and picking up some trashy Little Debbie snack cakes. A brilliant move, in my opinion.

My God, it all felt so freeing to just say no! Here's how it went down:

The morning of the school bake sale, I skipped out of the grocery store carrying twenty dollars' worth of heart-shaped snack cakes and felt like Mom of the Year. When I handed the bag to Stella, she looked at me with her big, beautiful, honey-colored eyes and said, "But Mommy, Anna's mom always makes homemade cookies."

Pre-hospital stay, that comment would have sent me down a shame spiral for not being the "kind of mom" who works all day and then stays up until midnight baking cookies. And honestly, if that's what she really *wanted* to do, then good for Anna's mom. What I really wanted to do the night before the bake sale was snuggle with my girls on the couch after dinner and be in bed by 9 p.m. So that's what I did, and it felt amazing.

I turned around and looked at Stella's sweet little face. I told her I loved her and her sister more than anything in the world and then gave her a kiss on her chubby little cheek. She giggled and didn't give the cookies another thought, and neither did I.

The guilt didn't come like it would have before because I did what was best for me at that moment. I'm really grateful that Anna's mom made homemade cookies, but the truth is I'm just not that mom. And that's okay.

I am the kind of mom who shows up and has hard conversations with my girls. I'm the kind of mom who will kiss every single boo-boo, both physical and emotional. I will advocate like a mama bear for my girls and love them with every fiber of my being. But let's be clear—I will never bake another goddamn cookie for a baked sale again when my gal pal Little Debbie can do it for me. Not my journey, sis, not my journey.

And the cherry on top of this whole story is that when I got home from work that evening, Stella ran up to me and was so proud to share that those damn Little Debbie's sold out first! Boundaries for the win! I didn't lead the bake sale... hell, I didn't even *bake* for the bake sale, and the world didn't fall apart. Quite the contrary...I got the rest and balance I needed, and Stella got some major first-grader street cred. It was a guilt-free win/win situation all the way around.

This might seem like a silly example, but the distinction between pre- and post–hospital stay is important to recognize. Pre-hospital stay, my health was such a non-priority that I let guilt and the need for acceptance trump my need for rest and balance. Prior to the near-ostomy-bag scare, I would never have quit a stable job or sent my kid to a school function with four boxes of premade, prepackaged treats because I would have felt I *should* have stayed in a job that made me miserable and that I *should be* the kind of mom who gave Martha Stewart a run for her money.

"Should" versus "want" is an important distinction. I challenge you to notice the next time you're asked to do something, to pause and ask yourself, "Do I really want to do this?" And if the answer is no, what's at stake if you politely decline? Sometimes you may come up with a perfectly valid answer. Sometimes you have to do something you don't necessarily want to because it's important to someone you love and doesn't compromise your own wants, needs, or health. But most of the time, what I think you'll find is that you're saying yes when all you really want to say is no.

It's OK to say no in favor of rest.

It's OK to say no in favor of balance.

It's OK to say no for no goddamn reason at all!

I'm not going to lie—this is still really hard for me. I still want to say yes or explain every single no I say—but practice and time have made it easier—especially when I remember what is at stake. No resentful "yes" will ever be worth my physical, mental, or emotional health ever again.

"No resentful 'yes' will ever be worth my physical, mental, or emotional health ever again."

CHAPTER 19

TRIPOD

———

Once I started making healthy changes like waking up and surrendering, noticing the lump, and setting boundaries, the next thing I needed to do was start taking responsibility for the role I played in managing my health. While it's not my fault I have a chronic illness, it is my responsibility to properly manage what is in my power to control.

I kept coming back to three key elements that, when left unchecked, typically led to worsening symptoms or a flare-up. The image of a tripod popped into my head with medication on one side, mental and emotional health on the second, and real self-care on the third. My remission and wellness balanced on the top of this imaginary tripod—and the moment one of the legs became weak or imbalanced, I would start to have symptoms.

At twenty-nine years old, all three sides were so unsteady and busted—of course, I came crashing down! There was nothing beneath me to support and hold me upright. Looking back, it happened that way every single time.

Taking responsibility for my health required brutal honesty with myself. For example, consistently working twelve-hour days, eating garbage, sneaking the occasional cigarette, not following up with regular doctor visits, and shoving down every difficult emotion was *clearly* not the way to handle this thing.

What I needed was a Remission and Wellness Tripod, so I drew one in my journal and committed myself to balance and daily check-ins. Here's how it works:

TRIPOD LEG #1: MEDICATION:

I'm no doctor, but apparently, medication doesn't work unless you take it as prescribed. Duh, right? It's not like I didn't *know* that; I just didn't *want* to know that. Why? A few reasons, really.

First of all, it was easy to fool myself into thinking skipping a day, or two, of medication, was no big deal. Or forgetting to get it refilled for an entire week.

Plus, some types of medication can have scary side effects. After I got out of the hospital, my doctor came up with a treatment plan (one that didn't include the loss of my rectum) and prescribed a medication called 6-MP. 6-MP (Mercaptopurine) is a chemotherapy drug with an increased risk of lymphoma and other cancers, pancreatitis (been there, done that!), and liver damage—just to name a few.

Taking this medication was a big mental hurdle for me to get over. I felt like I was putting poison in my body every single day. And the anxiety I felt having to choose between this type of medication and surgery was all-encompassing. I wondered, was I avoiding surgery in the short term, only to create another health issue in the long term?

Secondly, medication can be really expensive—and I thought if I stretched out my pills, I was actually being economical. (Tell that to my four-thousand-dollar hospital bill!)

I'm fortunate that the medication I take is fairly affordable with insurance.

However, there was a period of time when my insurance switched, and my medication wasn't covered until I hit a very high deductible. Imagine my surprise when I rolled up to the CVS drive-thru and was told the cost of my medication would be $1,500 when the month prior, it was less than a hundred dollars! CVS isn't in the business of financing medication payments, so I either had to pay in full or leave without the medication I needed to be healthy. At the time, that was more than my monthly house payment. So, with a pit in my stomach, I reluctantly handed over my credit card. What else could I do?

And I'm one of the lucky ones when it comes to medication costs. My friend's husband has Crohn's, and I was told that, without insurance, the price of a single infusion treatment was around twenty thousand dollars. With insurance, they paid $2,500 every eight weeks before the cost eventually came down years later.

The cost of medication in this country is a topic for another day and another book. But suffice it to say, it's an issue for millions of people in this country ... *the richest country in the world*. With or without insurance, the financial burden many people with chronic illness face is staggering. But we need our medication to thrive—and, for some people, to survive. So, we do what we need to do and take the financial hit.

And finally, when I wasn't flaring, taking medication seemed unnecessary ... especially considering the cost and potential side effects. This line of thinking, while very seductive, is dangerous. I had to realize—whether I was in remission or not—I needed to take my medication every day, as prescribed. It was that or surgery. The choice was mine and mine alone.

There's just something about taking medication every single day for the rest of one's life that can be a tough mental hurdle to get over. I get it; trust me, I do. It sucks. It's annoying. It can be expensive. But my friend, I say this with great love and kindness: *Get the fuck over it.*

Take your damn meds, whether you feel sick or not. Whether you want to or not. Whether they're expensive or not. If you can't afford your medication, there are many programs that can help defray the cost. And if, for some reason, you're experiencing negative side effects, please speak with your doctor and come up with a plan together. Trust me, you will do more damage in the long run if you don't get this side of the tripod set up and stable.

CYA Alert: I am not a doctor. Always seek the advice of your physician or other qualified health providers with questions regarding medication and treatment.

TRIPOD LEG #2: MENTAL & EMOTIONAL HEALTH:

I recently spoke with Dr. Tiffany Taft, a licensed clinical psychologist specializing in the psychological impacts of chronic digestive diseases. Dr. Taft also has Crohn's disease and is a total badass, clinician, researcher, advocate, and mom.

One day, she was speaking with a gastro who started to notice some of his patients exhibiting symptoms of PTSD. Dr. Taft was intrigued and decided to see what research existed on the topic of IBD and posttraumatic stress. She was surprised to find there were no studies in the United States on the subject. So, Dr. Taft decided to conduct her own research. (Badass, right?)

In her first research study on the topic, Dr. Taft compared patients with Inflammatory Bowel Disease (i.e., Crohn's and Ulcerative Colitis) to people with Irritable Bowel Syndrome—two very different gastrointestinal disorders. IBD is classified as a disease that causes destructive inflammation, permanent damage, is more likely to lead to surgery, and carries an increased risk of colon cancer. IBS is classified as a syndrome that does not cause inflammation, rarely leads to surgery, and is not associated with a higher risk of colon cancer. However, the bowel symptoms of IBD and IBS can be similar in a lot of people.

When she compared the test group (IBD patients) versus the control group (IBS patients), she found that 32 percent of IBD patients reported significant symptoms of posttraumatic stress—which are generally grouped into four categories:

- Intrusive memories
- Avoidance (my personal favorite, clearly)
- Negative changes in mood or thinking
- Changes in physical and emotional reactions

In her second study, she measured PTSD symptoms in almost eight hundred patients registered with the Crohn's & Colitis Foundation/University of North Carolina IBD Partners registry. Similar rates of PTSD symptoms existed—with women, and racial and ethnic minorities, reporting even higher rates of these symptoms than men or White patients. In almost one thousand IBD patients, 25–30 percent have significant PTSD due to their IBD experiences.

In the third study, Dr. Taft and her team interviewed around twenty patients with IBD to really understand what it is about IBD experiences that can be traumatic. The most dominant theme patients talked about was poor communication and information exchange between doctors and patients. A common scenario was a patient in the hospital for a major flare-up and a surgeon coming by to discuss surgical options—without addressing questions or anxieties.

Another common theme was trauma from nasogastric tubes, used to treat a bowel obstruction. These were described as torture, even leading one patient to describe considering suicide. While these are only a few studies, they clearly demonstrate the need for ongoing research and education regarding the intersection of mental health and chronic illness in the US. Not just because it exists and needs to be addressed, but because ongoing stress and anxiety actually impact physical health as well.

According to the *2019 Annual Report* published by the Crohn's & Colitis Foundation, a study conducted at the David Geffen School of Medicine found that patients with ulcerative colitis who experienced higher stress and anxiety were "significantly more likely" to experience a clinical flare-up.

Groundbreaking, I know.

One of the researchers from the study went on to say, "Anecdotally, patients report that stress makes their symptoms worse. We now have data to support that."

Well, congratu-fucking-lations, you now have your fancy data to support what millions of patients have known since the beginning of time. Bravo! Now, what are we actually going to do about it?

Long story short, not much. While there is a growing amount of support and research for the biopsychosocial aspects of chronic illness, unfortunately, many doctors still do not consider mental and emotional health as part of their treatment plan with patients. There are some amazing doctors who do—but unfortunately, it's not the norm. Until that changes, it's up to patients and badasses like Dr. Taft to advocate and shine a light on this important part of the Remission and Wellness Tripod.

Personally, the number-one trigger of a flare-up for me is stress. When my mental and emotional health aren't being managed, you can bet your rectum a flare-up isn't far behind. And because I never learned healthy coping mechanisms to deal with stress, I needed to teach myself. Here are a few of my favorite tips:

MEDICATION & THERAPY.

According to the Crohn's and Colitis Foundation, "Rates of depression are higher among patients with Crohn's disease and ulcerative colitis as compared to other diseases and the general population. Anxiety is also common in IBD patients." I know what you're thinking ... I already take enough medication; do I really need to take one more pill? Maybe not. Maybe you have a better tolerance for stress and anxiety. Maybe therapy is enough for you, or maybe stress doesn't impact your life and health like it does mine.

For me, anti-anxiety medication is part of my plan of care for managing Crohn's. I tried for years to pretend like I didn't need medication for my mental health, and guess what always ended up happening ... I'd get super stressed and anxious and eventually have a flare-up. I've been on and off SSRIs and in and out of therapy since I was nineteen, and this is what I know for sure: for me—ongoing therapy and medication increase my chances of staying in remission.

ENJOY THE RIDE.

Turns out, the therapist from my freshman year in college was right—exercise is a really good way to deal with stress and anxiety. Unfortunately, it took me years to learn that, because for me, exercise was always a means to an end—thinness. As someone who had an eating disorder, exercise has always been tricky for me, and I can slip into an unhealthy obsession pretty quickly. That is—until I discovered spin.

The first spin class I ever took was a disaster. I showed up with all of my old emotional baggage and worked out so hard I thought I might actually die or, at the very least, have a heart attack. I got home that evening and fell asleep at 7:30 p.m. in my sweaty workout clothes. I was terrified to go back but had purchased a three-pack and didn't want to waste it.

Before my second class, Joe gently suggested I take it easy this time around. "Maybe don't even worry about your stats or where you place on the leaderboard. Just show up and enjoy the ride."

I considered Joe's advice as I was warming up before class. But as soon as I sat on the bike, my heart started pounding with fear ... *Oh shit, this is going to hurt.* But did it have to? Did I have to push myself so hard? What if I stopped putting so much pressure on myself to burn a certain number of calories or come in first place—and just had fun?

So that's exactly what I did. I let go and had my own personal dance party on the bike. I didn't care how silly I looked, what noises I made, or what place I came in.

Then the instructor, a beautiful woman named Tracy, said something I'll never forget. "If you came here today to punish yourself for something you ate or did, you are missing the point. We do not exercise to punish ourselves; we exercise to reward ourselves!"

Whhhhaaat? Exercise as a reward?

"Your body was made to move and feel good! You deserve to celebrate that, and you are stronger than you realize!" Tracy shouted from the podium in front of the class.

Wait, my body was *made to feel good*? For as long as I could remember, my body was made to be two things: thin and defective. Or at least that's some bullshit I told myself years ago.

During the final acceleration of class, I did something I hadn't during the first class or up until that moment. I looked at myself in the wall-to-wall mirror in front of me and what I saw made me cry. I saw a woman who was healthy enough to exercise. I saw a woman who was having fun and enjoying the moment. I saw a woman whose body had the potential to be more than thin or ravaged by illness. I saw a woman who actually loved herself.

After that class, I decided to give myself the gift of exercise and committed to going to spin class three times a week to keep my tripod strong.

A few months later, I had been going through a rough patch at work, and prior to discovering the mental and emotional benefits of exercise, my coping mechanism was wine. And while I love me a big, bold glass of red wine, let's be honest, it's just another hiding place.

Instead of coming home from work and opening a bottle of wine, I would immediately swap my high heels for spin shoes and find joy riding on a stationary bike in a dark room—among strangers who would eventually become friends, while belting out P!nk at the top of my lungs. (Damn right, I Am Here!)

There were classes I would pray the entire time. There were other classes I'd cry big, ugly, snotty sobs. There were times I came in first place and times I came in last. None of it mattered because, for the first time in my entire life, I found a healthy way to cope with stress. One that made me physically, mentally, and emotionally stronger. You can't say that about a Cabernet Sauvignon.

TRIPOD LEG #3: *REAL* SELF-CARE:

The term "self-care" has become a super buzzy phrase over the last few years. I'm glad we've normalized taking better care of ourselves because the whole *who-can-burn-out-fastest* game is getting pretty tiring. However, I believe there is a difference between what I refer to as "Instagram Self-Care" and "Real Self-Care." You can typically tell the difference between the two if someone is making a profit.

And while treating yourself to a manicure is great, and I wholeheartedly support people making money ... that's not what I'm talking about as part of the third and final leg of the tripod.

I'm talking about the importance of rest, nutrition, and connection. Let's explore:

REST.

As I've already mentioned, one of the side effects of many autoimmune diseases is fatigue. The fatigue that accompanies chronic illness can be crippling, especially if left unchecked. Before I set up my Remission & Wellness Tripod, I rarely ever napped. I downright refused to because I had a mental list of all these things I just *had* to do. After I got out of the hospital in 2009, I committed myself to better rest and discovered the exquisite art of napping.

Holy moly! When was the last time you took an actual nap ... like ... at 2 p.m. on a Saturday afternoon? Or how about this move (one of my personal favorites): a midday power nap on a random weekday? Girl, I know you have a day job ... so do I! Here's how I do it:

On days when the fatigue is particularly heavy, I head to my car during my lunch break, lock the doors, set the alarm on my phone for forty minutes, turn on NPR, and let Rachel Martin lull me to sleep.

My sister thinks I'm insane for doing this, but you got to get in where you fit in, and those power naps give me LIFE! Sometimes I fall asleep, and other times I just close my eyes and rest. Either way, I always end up feeling better because I stepped away from the hustle and bustle of my job just long enough for a little mini self-care session in the form of rest.

I also used to fight going to bed early ... especially on the weekends. I would want to stay up late after running around all day and then feel like garbage as a result of not going to bed at a decent hour. Or friends would invite us over on a Friday night for dinner, and I felt rude saying I didn't want to go because I was tired.

Chronic disease or not, proper rest is vital for good health. If a friend thinks I'm lame because I'm choosing my well-being over a Friday night bonfire, then I guess they'll just have to just be disappointed. Life goes on, and from here on out, I will be well-rested in order to keep my Remission and Wellness Tripod balanced.

NUTRITION.

I almost typed the word "diet," but that word carries too much baggage, so I decided against it. When I was in my pre-hospital-denial phase, I was really hardheaded about food. I figured that no matter what I ate, I was going to get sick, so I might as well eat whatever the hell I wanted to.

Not a great plan.

Everyone's body responds to food differently, and there are lots of different food plans recommended for people with IBD and autoimmune disease. These types of programs work really well for some people. Unfortunately, for me, they don't; because anything remotely resembling a diet tends to trigger disordered eating. It's frustrating and something I still work on with my therapist to this day. (See Tripod #2.)

Instead of a limiting or strict diet, I try being mindful of how the food I consume makes me feel. For example, how does Diet Coke or a handful of Doritos make my body feel when I eat it? Nine times out of ten, the answer is usually "not so great." Those foods (I use the term loosely) usually make my stomach get super bloated and hurt. Does that mean I never have a Diet Coke or cheesy orange dust-covered fingers? No. But I limit those types of highly processed, chemically filled snacks as much as possible in favor of foods that do not come in a box, bag, or can.

Some days I do great, other days not even close, but I always come back to my body and how it *feels*. When I'm not flaring, I love to eat big salads with forty-seven different toppings. I also love to eat ice cream and drink coffee. When I am flaring, any of those three items will have me doubled over with pain and sprinting to the bathroom. So, I back off and give my colon as much rest as possible. For me, good nutrition and mindful eating is another way I practice Real Self-Care.

CONNECTION.

Connection with self and others is the last piece of Real Self-Care I will talk about. Human beings are hardwired for connection. Once I got out of the hospital, I realized that I wasn't making time for myself or others in any real, meaningful way.

Because I said yes to everything, I always felt rushed and distracted. So even if I was with a friend or family member, I wasn't fully present or necessarily enjoying the moment. Once I slowed down and stopped saying yes to everything,

I created more time and space for real, meaningful connections with myself and with others. I started reading and journaling again. I started prioritizing spending time with those I felt safe with and started eliminating toxic people from my life. This was really hard for me at first but got easier the more I practiced and remembered to approach myself—and the people in my life—with honesty.

While the Remission and Wellness Tripod may not stave off every flare-up or protect me from surgery, I knew it gave me a fighting chance, and was the best way I could care for and befriend my body and spirit. I also knew that I could look at myself in the mirror and tell the woman staring back at me that I loved her enough to at least try and exhaust all options. She is worth it. And so are you.

"Because I never learned healthy coping mechanisms to deal with stress, I needed to teach myself."

CHAPTER 20

WE GOT YOU

Once I committed myself to balance à la the Remission and Wellness Tripod, it was amazing how much better I felt physically and mentally and how much more fulfilling my personal and professional life became.

I spent the next five years watching my babies grow into the sweetest little fairies in the world and reconnecting with Joe, my friends, and my family. I also grew into my new job and felt like I was finally channeling my inner Angela Bower.

Then, I got a promotion; that scared the hell out of me, and all of my precious balance went out the window—and with it, my remission. The more intense the work became, the more I slipped back into my old ways, and within a few months, each leg of the tripod started to get rickety and wobbly. The blood, pain, and urgency I had nearly forgotten about returned with a vengeance.

When it comes to work, I've always struggled with just how much to disclose about my Crohn's. It's complicated, though—because when I'm flaring, my behavior can change. For instance, I might be in the middle of a one-on-one meeting with someone, and then all of a sudden feel a rumble from down-under and need to immediately leave and hightail it to the nearest restroom—which can seem a little strange without context.

The legal answer is that I don't have to tell anyone about anything. But what if I wanted to? What if I arrived at a place where I wasn't ashamed or scared to bring my whole self to work?

For a long time, I was afraid to say too much for fear people would think I was weak, not dependable, or not worthy of a promotion. For the first sixteen years of my career, the only time I took off work because of my Crohn's was either because I had a colonoscopy, or the week I spent in the hospital back in 2009. And even then, lying in a hospital bed, I begged my husband to bring me my cell phone and laptop. He refused and said I might want to get my head examined while I was in the hospital if I thought he was going to do that. Fair enough.

Then, a few years ago, I was sitting in a quarterly business review with various executives and my boss. After the meeting, my boss asked to speak with me.

"Christine, do you have a minute?"

I had stayed in my seat while everyone shuffled out of the conference room because I was in so much pain and was afraid that if I stood up, I would either pass out or shit my pants. Either way, not a great look.

Early that morning, it took every ounce of energy I had to get out of bed, shower, dress, put on makeup, and drive to work. In fact, I had to make an emergency stop on the way to work because I was so sick and knew there was no way I was going to make it the rest of the drive. Once I arrived at work, I proceeded to get sick another four times before the meeting took place.

"You really need to work on your poker face. You looked irritated the entire meeting, and that's just not like you. Everything okay?" my boss asked.

To tell or not to tell?

At the time, I was working on a team responsible for our largest, most challenging customer. We were a tight group that traveled together every month. We were a dedicated, passionate group of professionals who wanted to succeed and agreed it was the "hardest job we ever loved." I was also actively talking with my boss about a new position—and I didn't want to jeopardize my chance of getting a promotion.

It would have been easy to apologize for the miscommunication and shrug off his observation with the old standby, "I'm fine." But I didn't want my boss, who I greatly respected, to think I was being rude or unprofessional. I also trusted him as a leader and felt I could be honest with him. So, I took a deep breath and asked if he had a minute to talk.

"I know I've mentioned before that I have a pretty sensitive stomach. But the truth is, it's more than that. I have something called Crohn's disease, and I'm starting to have a flare-up. I apologize if I looked irritated, but the truth is, I was in so much pain at one point during the meeting, and didn't want to be disruptive and leave—so I just sat there and tried to manage through it." There it was. I told the truth. The cat was out of the bag, and there was no taking it back.

My boss could have brushed me off or told me to button it up, regardless of how I was feeling ... but he didn't. He leaned in from across the table and asked if I felt comfortable educating him on what exactly that meant so he could best support me. His sincerity took me a little off guard. He wasn't mad or disappointed; he was empathetic and curious—the hallmarks of a great leader who cares about the people on his team as much as the bottom line.

I told him what I was experiencing, even though it felt really awkward to say things like "urgency" in front of my boss. I told him I was unable to eat or drink much of anything, and if I did, I would immediately get sick.

I started to feel self-conscious after sharing such personal details. "But I'm okay. I promise I won't let this affect my work. I've worked through many flare-ups before, and I'm 100 percent committed to this team and doing whatever needs to be done. I promise, you can count on me."

He looked me in the eye and said something to the effect of, "I know I can count on you. That's why you're part of this team, and I greatly value your contributions. But what I need you to do right now is take care of yourself."

I tried to interrupt, but he wasn't having it.

"Honestly, you don't look well. I want you to go home and do what you need to feel better. Get in touch with your doctor, and once you have a plan, let me know and we'll go from there," he said. Then he said something I'll never forget: "We got you."

We got you.

Those three words meant the world to me. And the best part is, he actually meant it.

I ended up taking the remainder of the week off. My doctor prescribed a short dose of Prednisone and suggested I stick to clear liquids for the next few days to see if we could get things to calm down.

It was the first time I let myself fully tell the truth at work, and guess what ... the world didn't fall apart. And because I actually took the time to rest and follow my doctor's orders, my flare-up didn't spin out of control as it had years earlier.

I realize I was really lucky to work for such an understanding and thoughtful leader. Not everyone has that kind of relationship with their boss. The key is that I felt comfortable and safe sharing something so personal with him because of the relationship we'd built over the prior year. He was discreet, never brought it up in front of others, and didn't judge me for needing to take care of myself for a few days. In fact, a few months later, I got that promotion and felt healthier and stronger than I had in a long time because I didn't downplay or ignore what my body was trying to tell me. In the past, I would have let those symptoms go on for months before even calling my doctor. But because I faced my symptoms head-on, things were much more controllable this time around.

I can honestly say that having Crohn's disease made me a more compassionate human and leader. I learned from a young age that you just never know what someone else is going through. But, having a chronic illness means you typically pick up on the pain or discomfort of others pretty easily.

A few years ago, I was in a meeting with three women on my team when I could tell one woman wasn't feeling well. By this time, I had become very comfortable discussing my Crohn's and even the emotional challenges that accompany it. What did I have to hide? By that point, I had been promoted again—to my dream job with a dream team—and I wanted to create the same sense of safety that my prior boss created for me.

"Okay, let's get started," said the woman who I could tell wasn't feeling well, looking down at her notebook.

"Hold on ... what's going on?" I asked.

"Nothing. I'm fine," she said through tears.

There it was ... the biggest lie.

"Okay, meeting over." I shut my laptop. "Whatever we had to discuss at this meeting can wait."

And just as my boss had done for me years earlier, I leaned in and asked her what she needed and how I could help. I asked if she wanted to talk about whatever was upsetting her or if she preferred to be alone.

She wanted to talk and shared that she was feeling really stressed lately at home and work, then apologized for letting it get the best of her. We all listened and held space for her vulnerability. This space created room for the other women to open up and share their own concerns and struggles. I thanked them for all sharing how they felt and let them know I was feeling it too.

It would have been easy for me to ignore my teammate and take her response at face value. It would have been easy to forge ahead ... it's work, after all, not some group therapy session. But I would have missed the opportunity to build trust and learn more about what my team needed to be successful.

I asked a few more clarifying questions, and—as a team—we devised a plan to reshuffle some priorities.

Before leaving the room, the woman on my team who was feeling stressed thanked me for "being human" and allowing her to be as well.

I smiled and let her know the pleasure was all mine. Then I reassured her the best I knew how with the same words that brought me so much comfort when I was going through a tough time: "We got you."

"It was the first time I let myself fully tell the truth at work, and guess what ... the world didn't fall apart."

CHAPTER 21

CHRONIC COMPLAINERS

———

Did you know, on average, it can take four to five years to receive an accurate autoimmune disease diagnosis? Remember, nearly 80 percent of people living with autoimmune diseases are women. This most certainly is a women's health issue, and I know the medical community can do better. How? By listening to their patients and reserving judgment (more on that in a moment).

As research for this book, I interviewed many women with a variety of autoimmune diseases and a common theme that emerged (besides the lack of discussion around mental and emotional health) was how long it took to get an actual diagnosis.

I recently spoke with a family friend who, after decades of struggling with pain, fatigue, urgency, and diarrhea, was finally diagnosed with Crohn's disease at the age of sixty-six. For context, most people get diagnosed in their late teens or early twenties. She described multiple trips to the ER and how frustrated she felt because, for years, she knew deep down that something more was wrong. She was right.

That same week a childhood friend reached out to me with some questions about various symptoms she was having as a result of her IBS diagnosis. She described pain, urgency, frequency, flared joints, and the presence of mucous in her stool. I asked if she was ever tested for Celiac, Crohn's, or Ulcerative Colitis. Her answers were no, no, and no. Apparently, her doctor is hesitant to even consider an IBD diagnosis because she's "heavy" and hasn't experienced "severe weight loss," which, by the way, is total and complete bullshit—people of all shapes, sizes, colors, and creeds get IBD.

The following week I spoke with a different woman named Cat, who had ongoing stomach pain, fatigue, and canker sores in her mouth for years. She went to her primary care doctor in June of 2020 with what she thought was a bladder infection. When her doctor noticed she lost forty-five pounds since her last visit, instead of being concerned, the doctor ... wait for it ... *congratulated her* for losing weight.

Cat showed her doctor the multiple canker sores that lined the inside of her mouth and described the extreme pain she was experiencing in her rectum, both of which are symptoms of Crohn's disease—especially when paired with unintended, rapid weight loss. Cat felt like something more was wrong, but her doctor brushed her off and sent her home with a prescription for antibiotics to treat a nonexistent bladder infection.

Later that week, Cat told her sister-in-law what she was going through, how terrible she still felt, and that the antibiotics weren't kicking in. Her sister-in-law was so worried about Cat that she immediately got her in to see a gastroenterologist where she worked.

After receiving a colonoscopy, Cat was immediately diagnosed with Crohn's disease. Apparently, she did not have hemorrhoids, but the most anal fissures the gastroenterologist had ever seen, along with a large vaginal fistula (both painful complications of Crohn's disease) that would immediately require surgery to repair. A vaginal fistula is an opening that connects to another organ (in Cat's case, her rectum), allowing stool to pass through the vagina.

Unfortunately, Cat's surgeon discovered her fistula was four centimeters big, and he would not be able to repair it surgically. When Cat woke up, she learned that due to the size of the fistula, the only way to heal it was to shut down her colon in the affected area. "We are going to have to give you a temporary ostomy bag." That was October 2020 ... a mere four months after her alleged bladder infection. Cat was left feeling stunned, overwhelmed, and wondering how in the world this could happen.

Did all these ladies just have a stroke of unfortunate luck? Their stories sounded vaguely familiar to my own in that it took a few tries to get a doctor to actually take their symptoms seriously. Upon receiving a diagnosis, the women I interviewed all told me that, looking back, they always knew something was wrong.

It's only in the looking back that we remember what we always knew and just forgot. We *know* our bodies. We *know* when something isn't right. We feel it deep within our bones, and it's not until someone brushes us off or dismisses us that we start to second-guess ourselves.

Turns out dismissing women in pain is nothing new. I was curious to better understand this phenomenon and discovered a few nuggets I honestly didn't realize before I started writing this book. I want you to remember these "fun facts" the next time anyone in the medical community tries to brush you, a friend, daughter, sister, or partner and her symptoms off.

"FUN FACT" #1

According to a study conducted by the American Auto-immune Related Diseases Association, over half of the people with an autoimmune disease will see an average of four doctors. According to the same study, almost half of women were first labeled as "chronic complainers" by their physician prior to receiving an autoimmune disease diagnosis.

I often wonder what happened to those women who weren't labeled as "chronic complainers." Are they still suffering in silence? How much worse have their symptoms become?

"FUN FACT" #2

Women are less likely to receive aggressive treatment when diagnosed with pain but are more likely to have their pain be dismissed as "emotional" or "not real."

This one really frosts my cookies and reminds me of when I was in labor with my second daughter, Roma. When I arrived at the hospital, I knew I was in the late stages of labor by the level of pain I was experiencing. Plus, I had delivered my oldest daughter, Stella, only two hours after I arrived at the hospital and knew my body labored quickly.

God bless the triage nurses at the hospital. They were sweet as pie but slow as molasses. I heard them talking, and no one believed I was as far along as I *knew* I was. The pain was rapidly increasing, and I struggled to change out of my clothes and into a hospital gown between contractions.

"Excuse me ... can someone please check and see how dilated I am?" I tried to sound polite but felt like my body was being ripped apart.

Figuring they knew my body better than I did, no one was in a rush to examine me, even though I was writhing in pain. A nurse finally came in, took her time putting on a pair of latex gloves, and performed a pelvic exam. Within seconds, I heard her say, "Oh boy!"

"Oh boy—*what*?" I whispered through contractions.

"You're nine centimeters dilated!" She sounded a little panicky. "We need to get you into a labor and delivery room right now!"

My first thought was, "I told you so." My second thought was, "Somebody better get the lady with the epidural on the horn and have her meet us in the delivery room ASAP!"

"Oh honey, it's too late to get an epidural," one of the nurses said to me.

By then, I was a little older and a little wiser and wasn't about to be dismissed. "If we aren't in the delivery room yet, it's not too late. This is my body and my birth, and I want an epidural. I've been here before, and I know how this works. Someone needs to call the anesthesiologist immediately and tell her to meet us in the delivery room. The moment we get there, you—or someone—needs to start my IV, or else she won't be able to give me the epidural. It's not too late, and that's what I want."

And guess what? I got the dang epidural. But had I been too shy or too polite to speak up and advocate for myself in that moment, I would not have received any pain management. And while I wholeheartedly applaud women who give birth without any drugs ... I am not one of those women. In that moment, I became a woman who advocated for her body and medical care. The lesson I learned on that day was to speak up or suffer in pain.

"FUN FACT" #3

Even though over 30 percent of people living with Crohn's disease report experiencing post-traumatic stress, there is no standard for mental health screening as part of a routine examination. In addition to increased post-traumatic stress, according to WebMD, people with chronic illness also report higher levels of depression and anxiety; and are more likely to develop an eating disorder ... especially people with IBD.

For the life of me, I can't figure out why mental health screenings aren't the standard practice of care. They test and screen us for everything else. They test our blood and our stool. They examine our rectums and colons. They poke and prod us top to bottom. They examine everything ... except our minds.

As soon as my daughters turned twelve years old, they started to get a depression screening as part of their annual well visits. Why not do the same for people with chronic illness? Between the medication, doctor visits, battles with insurance companies, and medical bills—and then the actual disease itself—I would think some form of mental health screening is more than valid. What's baffling to me about all of this is that science has proven the brain-gut connection and the negative impact stress can have on symptoms.

I know for a fact, the years I was the sickest were the years I was most anxious and stressed. My doctor never talked to me about stress management or effective therapies and strategies to manage and care for my mental health or, at the very least, make a referral to someone who could help.

According to Dr. Megan Riehl, a prominent GI psychologist at the University of Michigan, the brain and gut are constantly communicating. Dr. Riehl works with her patients using evidence-based brain-gut treatments that target GI motility (the movement of food through the body) and abdominal pain. She also helps her patients with stress management and healthy ways to cope ... something most of us were never taught. (Sweet Jesus, where was Dr. Riehl when I was first diagnosed?)

When I asked Dr. Riehl why specialists don't discuss or refer their patients to mental health professionals as a standard practice, she told me the reason is pretty simple: "More education and advocacy need to be done."

Challenge accepted!

I don't know about you, but I'm a pretty impatient lady. I don't want to wait for these discussions to be part of the standard practice of care. So, it's up to us, the patients, to educate our doctors. Imagine the collective power we have if every person with a chronic illness spoke candidly about how mental and emotional health affects their physical symptoms. The more doctors hear the same message over and over again directly from patients, the better chance we have to impact change. So, if you feel comfortable doing so— please speak up! We can no longer talk about remission or symptom management without also talking about mental and emotional health.

I will now carefully step down from my soapbox and invite you to rethink the term *"chronic,"* once and for all.

"We can no longer talk about remission or symptom management without also talking about mental and emotional health."

CHAPTER 22

CHRONIC LOVE

———

Webster's Dictionary defines the word "chronic" as: "continuing or occurring again and again for a long time." The word "chronic" is also typically associated with negative things like disease, pain, and complainers. If we're going to become the best advocates we can for ourselves, I say it's time we reclaim this word! Let's identify what we will be positively chronic about so we might feel more empowered and in control. Remember what Glinda the Good Witch said ... we had the power all along.

CHRONIC TRUTH-TELLERS

Let's start by becoming chronic truth-tellers. We've already established that we aren't saying "I'm fine" anymore, right? This includes not just when family and friends ask but when our doctors ask, too. Especially when our doctors ask! I recently spoke to Dr. Aline Charabaty, the clinical director of gastroenterology and director of the Inflammatory Bowel Disease Center at Sibley Memorial Hospital. She told me the patients she worries most about are the ones who insist to her that they're fine. In her experience, those are the patients who often need the most help and care.

Dr. Charabaty's approach is to take a little more time with these patients, to ask more specific questions and help gently guide them to understand that maybe they aren't so fine—and that's okay. She goes on to say that the reason patients don't tell the truth to their medical team is that they're afraid to admit they're losing control. But, if we are afraid to admit we've lost control, we have no chance of regaining it.

Believe me, I know this type of chronic truth-telling is scary. No one wants to admit things have gotten worse for fear of what that might mean—another scope or scan, more aggressive treatment, a potential hospital stay, or surgery. But if we want to give our bodies the best shot of getting and staying healthy, we must be brave and tell the truth—in painstaking detail. Because lying about our physical, mental, and emotional health only leads to one place ... more pain, which is the very thing we're trying to avoid when we lie.

Being a chronic truth-teller requires a mix of bravery and vulnerability. I know it can feel overwhelming and scary at times, but as a yoga teacher once said to me in class, "What we resist, persists." I nearly fell over mid-tree pose when I heard this because it could be applied to so many areas of my life ... my health, especially. Every time I resisted calling my doctor at the first sight of blood or asking for help when I felt stressed or exhausted—things always got worse.

CHRONIC SUPPORT

"You're not alone" might be one of the most powerful things you can say to someone with a chronic condition or disease because often, it can feel so isolating. I interviewed so many women with IBD and other chronic illnesses for this book, and the one thing I heard from each and every one of them was how helpful it was to share their story with another person. For many of the women I spoke with, it was the first time they had done so since being diagnosed.

Finding healthy, ongoing support is another way we can advocate and care for ourselves. There is something so empowering about telling our story out loud to another person. In the right environment and with the right person, it can feel so freeing. I challenge you to give it a try sometime. I think you'll be surprised how you feel afterward. And bonus—this type of honest sharing often causes a ripple effect that leads to richer conversations and more meaningful connections with others. (Chronic support for the win!)

Once I finally started opening myself up to the Crohn's and Colitis community, I was surprised how much more informed I became as a patient—and how less alone I felt. If you are struggling with a chronic illness or condition of any kind, please seek support however you feel most comfortable. Support can come in the form of community, friendship, an incredible therapist, the right doctor, a partner, or a spouse.

The key to chronic support is that we must be open to receive it and then do so wholeheartedly. Support doesn't mean we are weak or troubling others with our problems (I've told myself that lie too many times). It means we are strong and dialed into caring for our precious bodies, hearts, and minds. And the best part about letting others in and accepting support is that you find yourself with advocates to walk beside you on your journey.

Did you know there is an entire community of people living with IBD out there waiting for you? These people are the brave warriors who've chosen to share their triumphs, heartaches, tips, and tricks with you when you're ready. It wasn't until recently that I started opening myself up to the IBD community, and I'm so glad I did. At the risk of dating myself, there was no such thing as Google, blogs, or social media when I was diagnosed. I can't even imagine how less alone I would have felt as a teenager, college student, young wife, mom, and professional—had I found this community sooner.

But the truth is, even if blogs and social media existed back then, I probably wouldn't have engaged. Heck, I didn't want to engage as early as five years ago! While I've typically been pretty open about my Crohn's on the surface—I never really wanted to talk about it with other people who also had Crohn's, other than my sister. Looking back, there were a few reasons why:

First, I didn't think I deserved to be part of the club. The strange part about Crohn's disease for me personally is that when I'm not having a flare-up, I almost forget that I even have a chronic illness. If it weren't for the handful of pills I take each day, the underlying fatigue, and the annual colonoscopy—it could be easy for me to pretend that I'm just like any other healthy person. It's not until I start flaring that everything starts to hit me all over again. It's not until things get so bad that I can't even take a sip of water without getting violently ill that I start to remember just how intense and serious this illness can be.

Also, unlike my sister, I've never had surgery. Unlike many of the incredible IBD warriors I've recently connected with, I don't have an ostomy bag. Although I share the same diagnosis, for years, I didn't feel I deserved to join the conversation. But here's the thing—it's not a competition for "Who can be the sickest?" or "Who's had the most surgeries or complications?" And while I can't know what it's like to live with an ostomy bag, I do know what it's like to feel sick, weak, overwhelmed, and scared about this disease. And from what I've experienced, no one even cares as long as you show up ready to respectfully listen, learn, and contribute in whatever way is best for you. This community needs more voices, more stories, and more warriors. Regardless of your particular symptoms and treatments, whether you're experiencing a flare or haven't flared in years—we all deserve the support and connection that comes from being part of a community.

Secondly, I was chicken shit. I was too afraid to acknowledge just how bad Crohn's could be and wasn't interested in seeing pictures of people in hospital beds, getting infusions, or in a bikini with their ostomy bag proudly on display. For so long, I wasn't ready to identify as someone who had a chronic illness. It was just another form of denial and burying my head in the sand. And while only you can know when you are ready, I would encourage you to dip your toe in the community pool, whatever your condition, sooner rather than later.

I'm not saying you have to follow every single person with the same condition as you on their socials or start a YouTube channel documenting a play-by-play account of your life. But maybe start by searching some hashtags, reading some posts, and seeing how you feel. Remember, listen to your body. If something isn't serving you, or you just aren't ready to see or read what someone else is posting about—that is 100 percent okay. Give yourself grace and move on.

Once I was ready to acknowledge there was a whole world of strong warriors out there, it actually had the exact opposite effect ... I felt less afraid. I saw all of these incredible women and men living their lives, educating themselves and others, advocating for better treatment and access to care, and lending support to their fellow "Crohnies." I saw firsthand that my greatest fear since I was diagnosed—getting a bag—was nothing to fear at all. I saw that I too could be strong, brave, and vulnerable, and if, God forbid, things got bad, there would be an entire community I could turn to for advice, support, and love.

CHRONIC CURIOSITY

In order to advocate for ourselves, we must also be chronically curious about ourselves. If it's been a while or you've never taken the time to really get to know yourself, what are you waiting for? Being chronically curious about yourself starts with a clear understanding of what makes you feel good and whole. It can be small things like a comfortable pair of sweats on a particularly bloated day. It can be a morning meditation followed by a warm shower with your favorite body wash. It could be river dancing to Lady Gaga, for all I care! The point is, if you don't know what makes you feel good, comforted, and loved—how will you make time for those things in your life? Being chronically curious and then dedicating time each day for yourself is the key to unlocking Real Self-Care.

On the flip side, getting curious about what doesn't make you feel good is equally important. For me, noticing how I feel around certain people is one way I've become more curious as I've gotten older. When I am around certain people, my body feels tense and tight. And as someone with a chronic illness, feeling tense and tight is what I need to avoid as much as possible. Notice how you feel around certain people and situations. Notice how certain foods or beverages make you feel. Notice how you feel when you don't give yourself permission to rest and recharge. Notice how you feel when someone doesn't respect a boundary you've set. Notice! Notice! Notice!

One of the best ways I've learned to advocate for myself is by getting chronically curious about what my body and spirit need and, conversely, what it cannot tolerate. Knowing my triggers helps me feel empowered to set and stick to healthy boundaries and not second-guess myself.

CHRONIC LOVE

And finally, perhaps the most important and powerful of all is chronic love. Our bodies—no matter how different or disabled—deserve love. They deserve love when they are in pain (*especially* when they're in pain) and when they feel like a million bucks. They deserve love when they feel mad and angry and when they feel happy and whole. Learning to love something within you that causes pain or anxiety is not easy. But let's remember, our bodies were created by the most powerful force in the Universe: *love*. And real, lasting comfort and healing depend on that same force.

* * *

Confession: I had a really hard time writing the end of this book because I found myself writing it from my "fancy airport woman" persona. Why? The recovering people-pleaser in me felt compelled to neatly wrap up the end and put a cute little bow on it for you. I really wanted to tell you that everything is going to be okay from here on out. Unfortunately, I can't do that.

I would be lying if I said the work of cultivating a chronically positive mindset is easy. It's not—far from it, actually. Like a beautiful garden, it requires time, patience, and tending. Weeds can quickly pop up and ruin the whole damn thing if you're not paying attention.

To this day, I still struggle with slowing down and probably always will. It's how I'm wired and part of what makes me who I am. It's taken years of self-reflection and practice to love myself enough to hold myself accountable when I start to slide back into old patterns of fear-based living. I still struggle with loving my body and wishing it were different. And I still struggle with feeling grief and anger about having a chronic illness: not because I don't accept it, but because I'm still a little afraid of it. *And that's okay.* It's entirely possible to fear something and nurture it at the same time. The key is to not let fear overshadow love.

While I can't wave a magic wand and take away my or your chronic illness or condition, I can tell you this: Keep trying and keep showing up for yourself every day, one day at a time. Get to know yourself—listen to your body and your feelings. Stop running away from the discomfort. Acknowledge it, explore it and feel it—all of it—the good, the bad, the embarrassing ... whatever. And when you start to feel the big feelings that come with a chronic illness or condition, please don't hide or hibernate. Beginning today, commit to setting up your own Remission and Wellness Tripod and then find someone (or group of someones) who will lovingly hold you accountable when things start to get shaky.

A Course in Miracles says nothing but love is real. Everything else is an illusion. When I remember that my anxiety and fear are illusions, it allows me to take a deep breath, bring myself back to the present moment—and remember that I am strong enough to face anything.

I'm not, never was, and never will be perfect. The miracle is that I no longer strive to be because perfection is an illusion, just like fear. I am a work in progress and will be until I take my last breath.

Are you ready to get started?

"Our bodies—no matter how different or disabled— deserve love."

PART 4 JOURNAL PROMPTS:

———

- What types of activities, situations, and people make you feel best physically, mentally, and emotionally? In what ways can you make *more* time and space for these in your life?
- What types of activities, situations, and people make you feel worse? In what ways can you make *less* time and space for these in your life?
- What does your Remission and Wellness Tripod consist of?

RESOURCES & OTHER COOL THINGS

———

WORRY IV NOTHING JOURNAL

The *Worry IV Nothing* journal is such an awesome tool that I have gifted to myself and others over and over again. My friend Ashley and her sister created this journal, which leverages techniques used in Cognitive Behavioral Therapy (CBT) after struggling with mounting anxiety during the early months of the COVID-19 shutdown. The journal helps to "document and deconstruct our automatic thoughts, teaching us to interpret and rebuild them in a more productive and accurate way." As I mentioned throughout the book, one of the greatest aspects of living with a chronic illness I personally struggle with is anxiety. And while there is no replacement for a great therapist—this journal has become a lifeline I use between therapy appointments when anxiety starts to build. I love to keep this discreet journal in my purse, so I have it with me should I fall into a "what-if" spiral. Visit fourprogress.com to learn more.

BOOKS

A Return to Love: Reflections on the Principles of "A Course in Miracles" by Marianne Williamson

The Choice: Embrace the Possible by Dr. Edith Eva Eger

The Body Is Not an Apology: The Power of Radical Self-Love by Sonya Renee Taylor

Set Boundaries, Find Peace: A Guide to Reclaiming Yourself by Nedra Glover Tawwab

The Power of Now: A Guide to Spiritual Enlightenment by Eckhart Tolle

The Gifts of Imperfection: Let Go of Who You Think You're Supposed to Be and Embrace Who You Are by Brene Brown

Playing Big: Practical Wisdom for Women Who Want to Speak Up, Create, and Lead by Tara Mohr

Untamed by Glennon Doyle

What Doesn't Kill You: A Life with Chronic Illness — Lessons from a Body in Revolt by Tessa Miller

PODCASTS

Unlocking Us with Brené Brown

We Can Do Hard Things with Glennon Doyle

Who Does She Think She Is? with Stephanie Llewelyn

iWeigh with Jameela Jamil

On Purpose with Jay Shetty

Girls with Guts with Alanna Martella & Nikki Dee

Uninvisible Pod with Lauren Freedman

Rule Breakers by Rebelle with Shannon Siriano Greenwood

QUOTES TO MAKE YOU THINK

"There is no illusion greater than fear." —Lao Tzu

"Hating our bodies is something that we learn, and it sure as hell is something that we can unlearn." —Megan Jayne Crabbe

"You can't heal what you don't feel." —Dr. Edith Eger

"Nothing changes if nothing changes." —Donna Barnes

"The ego is quite literally a fearful thought." —*A Course in Miracles*

"The moment of surrender is not when life is over. It's when it begins." —Marianne Williamson

"You are not upset for the reason you think. There is only one problem, choosing fear over love." —*A Course in Miracles*

"And I said to my body softly, 'I want to be your friend.' It took a long breath and replied, 'I have been waiting my whole life for this.'" —Nayyirah Waheed

"The quality of your recovery is proportional to the quality of your surrender." —(Unknown)

BLOGS & SOCIAL

There is power in connecting with others who are in a similar situation. That's why I created the "Chronic" Book Club Facebook Group early in my book-writing journey. The group is a place for women living with chronic illness of any kind looking to connect and learn from one another. I wanted a place women felt safe to ask questions and share experiences in an open and honest way without judgment. The only rule is you have to be respectful, kind, and honest. I hope you'll join us when and if you're ready!

If you have IBD (Crohn's or Ulcerative Colitis), there are many fantastic Facebook Groups and bloggers you might want to check out. Below are a few of my favorite:

CHRISTINE M. RICH

Come follow me on Instagram @christinerich_author or visit me online at christinemrich.com for more information.

GIRLS WITH GUTS PRIVATE FORUM: SUPPORT FOR WOMEN WITH IBD AND/OR OSTOMY

What's great about this group is that you can request a laminated "I Gotta Go!" medical emergency card, which can help you gain access to public restrooms as needed.

OWN YOUR CROHN'S: A COMMUNITY EMPOWERING SOUTH ASIANS WITH DIGESTIVE AILMENTS

I met Tina Aswani Omprakash (or, as I refer to her, "Tina the Fucking Warrior") when I was doing research for the book. Tina is a brilliant and brave advocate who works to normalize chronic illnesses and disabilities—with an emphasis on diversity and inclusion. Her jam is destigmatizing the shame that can shroud chronic disease. Her blog is full of incredible information and resources.

LIGHTS, CAMERA, CROHN'S

Natalie Hayden from *Lights, Camera, Crohn's* was the one who introduced me to "Tina the Fucking Warrior" and is also an amazing advocate who volunteers with the Crohn's & Colitis Foundation. Her blog is another terrific resource for those living with or loving someone with IBD.

ACKNOWLEDGEMENTS

I didn't know it then, but I started writing *Chronic* in my senior year at Kent State University, during a creative writing class taught by a brilliant professor named Maj Ragain. Maj and I started out on shaky ground—mostly because I was a jealous, immature writer who was so afraid of her own voice and story. Thankfully, we made amends by the end of the semester. One afternoon during office hours, we had words ... I apologized for the chip on my shoulder, and Maj made me realize what I was capable of as a writer if I could learn to trust myself and just let go. It only took me twenty years to get there. I wish I could send a copy of this book to Maj and personally thank him. Sadly, he passed away in 2018.

To my family—Thank you, Joe, Stella, and Roma, for your love, support, and encouragement. Thank you for your infinite patience and for putting up with every anxiety attack and mild tantrum I threw during the writing process. Thank you for not allowing me to stop when things got hard or uncomfortable. Thank you for giving me the space to write, process, and finally come to terms with my chronic illness. Thank you for your love—I am truly the luckiest wife and mother in the entire world because of you.

To my sister—Thank you for making me laugh harder than anyone in the entire world, for understanding firsthand the meaning of "rectal dry heaves," for loving me as I am and never thinking I'm too sensitive or too much. (Or, at least not saying it out loud!) Thank you for teaching me all the things that a big sister probably should have taught her little sister. Thank you for hearing and seeing me as very few people can. Baby sis, you are my heart.

To my best friends—Thank you, Michelle Persichetti and Kristin Garner, for all of the phone calls, text messages, words of wisdom, and encouragement. Thank you for holding space for me as I am and for always showing up. A thirty-year friendship is something to cherish—and I am beyond grateful to have such incredible women in my life. Thank you for being such a huge part of my story and for teaching me about things like bravery, boundaries, and self-love. I feel infinitely safe in our friendship—thank you, thank you, thank you, my soul sisters.

To Koren—Thank you for healing my spirit and helping me realize that it was never my fault.

To my parents—Thank you, Joe and Ann Bernard, for advocating for a diagnosis and for doing the best you could to love and support me throughout my life. Even though we rarely see eye-to-eye, I do love you both and am grateful for the sacrifices you made for me.

To my developmental editor—Thank you, Jackie Claire Reineri Calamia, for helping get my story out of my head and for pushing me to write as authentically as possible. Thank you for recognizing how vulnerable this content is and for treating it with the respect and tenderness it needed to grow.

To my marketing revisions editor—Thank you, Sandy Huffman, for helping me turn twenty-one chapters of content into something I love and am proud to share. Also, thank you for the belly laughs during our weekly calls and for helping me not take myself too seriously.

To the women who so generously shared their stories, expertise, and time with me—you ladies gave me the courage to keep writing and the strength to finally own my story. As I told Natalie Hayden, I may be late to the party, but I am here now with my party pants on! Thank you, Natalie Hayden, Tina Aswani Omprakash (aka Tina the Fucking Warrior), Shannon Siriano Greenwood, Kelly Fredrickson, Sharon Nivert, Jesse Miller, Jennie Persichetti, Leslie Sullivan, Catherine Marquard, Dixie Grace Bolton, Chealynn Feaster, Christina Owens, Dr. Megan Riehl, Dr. Aline Charabaty, Dr. Tiffany Taft and Janelle Paris. You are all amazing warriors and champions of women's physical, mental, and emotional health.

And finally, thank you to all of the people who supported the pre-sale campaign. Without your generosity, I could not have published *Chronic*. And for that, I am chronically grateful.

Abby Sullivan, Allison Jagunic, Allison Knecht, Amy Eagleeye, Ann Castellarin-Bianchi, Annie Lerman, Any McNair, April Murray, Ashley Hopkins-Shack, Babs Ryan, Beau Miller, Becky Meckstroth, Billy Roach, Bob Peel, Carol Miller, Cat Cook, Christy Kaprosy, Cindy Petrik, Kelly Jebber, Colleen Noffert, Crystal Sullivan, Dana Barna, Dana Pisani, Deanne Sprenger, Debbie Butler, Debra Parker, Debbie & Rocco Rich, Devin Hanley, Dina Edwards, Elizabeth Draeger, Emily Roggenburk, Eric Koester, Erin Loss, Francesca Nist, Hayley Kane, Helena Levesque, Kathryn Howells, Jackie Sullivan, Jaclyn Alter, Jaclyn Ruelle, Jamie LaDuca, Janelle Paris, Jenelle Maddox, Jennie Persichetti, Jessica Pundole, Jessica Weese, Joe & Ann Bernard, Joy Oldfield, Julie Gucciardo,

Julie Herceg, Justin Brazie, Katie Kapferer, Kelly Fredrickson, Kelly Parker, Kelsey & Adam Rich, Kevin Brainard, Kim Dalessandro, Kim McFarlane, Kim Simbeck, Koren Bierfeldt, Kristin Garner, Kristy Gierosky, Kylie Rambo, Laura Meyer, Lauren Krasnodembski, Lauren Persichetti, Lauren Smith, Lauren Yard, Lori Krohn, Mackenzie Finklea, Mandi Montgomery, Mandy Albaugh, Marcia Roach, Marra Pirtle, Mary Ann Maslar, Mary Jo Orr, Matt Garner, Meghan & Kirk Olmstead, Mindy Broerman, Melissa Coia, Michael & Ashley Goeren, Michelle Persichetti, Mike Chadsey, Miranda Castle, Nancy Awender, Nicole Watson, Noreen Hernan, Pamela Seiple, Patti & AJ Kraynack, Rachel Strnad, Randi Rich, Becca Murphy, Robbyn Watkins, Rose Mary Humble, Royce & Debbie Mitchell, Sally Woznicki, Samantha Testa, Sara Ruble, Sara Sadaghiani, Sarah McDaniel, Sarah Nicolaou, Sharon Nivert, Sharon Sullivan, Stacy Proskovec, Stefanie Perry, Stephanie Goldick, Tam Zawodny, Taryn Harrington, Teresa Norris, Todd Fennell, Tracy Richards, Valerie Geiger, Whitney Alter

APPENDIX (CHRONIC)

———

INTRODUCTION

- Watson, Stephanie. "Autoimmune Disease: Types, Symptoms, Causes and More." *Healthline*, March 2019. https://www. healthline.com/health/autoimmune-disorders.

CHAPTER 2

- Hayden, Natalie, "Putting the Debate to Rest: IBD Fatigue Isn't Your 'Normal' Type of Tired"; *Lights, Camera, Crohn's*; October 2020. https://lightscameracrohns.com/tag/fatigue.

CHAPTER 3

- Milligan, Susan. "The Value of Women." *U.S. News & World Report*, December 2017. https://www.usnews.com/news/the-report/articles/2017-12-05/study-women-valued-for-physical-attractiveness.

CHAPTER 6

- Psychology Today. "Grief: Bereavement." Accessed June 22, 2021. https://www.psychologytoday.com/us/basics/grief.

CHAPTER 14

- Williamson, Marianne. *A Return to Love: Reflections on the Principles of A Course in Miracles.* San Francisco: Harper One, 1996.

CHAPTER 15

- Taylor, Sonya Renee. *The Body Is Not an Apology: The Power of Radical Self-Love.* Oakland: Berrett-Koehler Publishers, 2020.

CHAPTER 19

- Hlavinka, Elizabeth. "Physiological Stress Measures Predict Ulcerative Colitis Flares—Unpacking the link between the brain and the microbiome." *MedPage Today,* January 2020. https://www.medpagetoday.com/meetingcoverage/ccc/84539.

- Taft, Tiffany H., Alyse Bedell, Meredith R. Craven, Livia Guadagnoli, Sarah Quinton, and Stephen B. Hanauer. Inflammatory Bowel Disease Patients. Inflammatory Bowel Diseases 25, no. 9 (August 2019): 1577-1585. Accessed June 24, 2021. doi: 10.1093/ibd/izz032. https://pubmed.ncbi.nlm.nih.gov/30840762.

- Taft, Tiffany H., Alyse Bedell, Meredith R. Craven, Livia Guadagnoli, Sarah Quinton, and Stephen B. Hanauer. "Initial Assessment of Post-traumatic Stress in a US Cohort of Inflammatory Bowel Disease Patients." Inflammatory Bowel

Diseases 25, no. 9 (September 2019): 1577–1585. Published online 2019 Mar 7. doi: 10.1093/ibd/izz032. https://www.ncbi.nlm.nih. gov/pmc/articles/PMC7534390/.

CHAPTER 21

- Brauser, Deborah. "Eating Disorders and Autoimmune Disease Linked." *WebMD*, September 2014. https://www. eatingdisorderhope.com/information/eating-disorder/ the-link-between-eating-disorders-and-autoimmune-disease.

- Rabbitt, Meghan. "Inside the Epidemic of Misdiagnosed Women"; *Prevention*, April 2020. https://www.prevention.com/ health/a32085516/common-misdiagnosis-women.